# THE HOLFORD
# 9-DAY LIVER DETOX

## Also by Patrick Holford

*The Holford Low-GL Diet*

*The Holford Low-GL Diet Made Easy*

*The Holford Diet GL Counter*

*Patrick Holford's New Optimum Nutrition Bible*

*Patrick Holford's New Optimum Nutrition for the Mind*

*Optimum Nutrition for Your Child's Mind* (with Deborah Colson)

*Food is Better Medicine than Drugs* (with Jerome Burne)

*500 Health and Nutrition Questions Answered*

*Hidden Food Allergies* (with Dr James Braly)

*The Alzheimer's Prevention Plan* (with Shane Heaton and Deborah Colson)

*The H Factor* (with Dr James Braly)

*Optimum Nutrition Before, During and After Pregnancy* (with Susannah Lawson)

*Boost Your Immune System* (with Jennifer Meek)

*Balancing Hormones Naturally* (with Kate Neil)

*The Optimum Nutrition Cookbook* (with Judy Ridgway)

*Solve Your Skin Problems* (with Natalie Savona)

*Beat Stress and Fatigue*

*Improve Your Digestion*

*Say No to Arthritis*

*Say No to Cancer*

*Say No to Heart Disease*

## Also by Patrick Holford and Fiona McDonald Joyce:

*The Holford Low-GL Diet Cookbook*

*Smart Food for Smart Kids*

# THE HOLFORD 9-DAY LIVER DETOX

## THE DEFINITIVE DIET THAT DELIVERS RESULTS

### PATRICK HOLFORD
### & FIONA McDONALD JOYCE

PIATKUS

First published in Great Britain in 2007 by Piatkus Books

A CIP catalogue record for this book
is available from the British Library

ISBN 978-0-7499-2755-4

Edited by Jan Cutler
Designed and typeset by Paul Saunders

Printed and bound in Great Britain by
MPG Books, Bodmin, Cornwall

Piatkus Books
An imprint of
Little, Brown Book Group
100 Victoria Embankment
London EC4Y 0DY

An Hachette Livre UK Company

www.piatkus.co.uk

# Acknowledgements

I would especially like to thank my wonderful co-author, Fiona, who is not only a great cook and nutritionist, but super-efficient! Also Rachel Nicoll and Virgina Harry for their help researching for this book, and Jo Brooks and Jan Cutler at Piatkus for their tireless editing. Most of all, thanks to my wife Gaby for her help and encouragement, for working around the clock, and to all the willing volunteers who tried and tested our 9-Day Liver Detox Diet.

*Patrick Holford*

# Contents

# PART ONE

# Introduction

Thirty years ago I was introduced to the concept that most common Western diseases were largely the result of less than perfect nutrition. Although I was sceptical to begin with, after two months on a diet packed with fresh fruit and vegetables and supported by nutritional supplements, I saw the evidence for myself: I looked well, felt great and had more vitality and mental clarity than ever before.

This experience was the beginning of a life-long journey that resulted in my founding The Institute for Optimum Nutrition (ION) in 1984, with the help and support of twice Nobel-prize-winner Dr Linus Pauling. ION, an independent non-profit-making educational charity, is now one of the leading schools in Europe for training nutritional therapists. Its purpose is to educate the public and health professionals about the importance of optimum nutrition through its own publications, educational courses and community outreach programmes. ION also advises people on nutritional therapy and offers treatment where necessary.

Over the years, I have travelled all over the world lecturing on nutrition as well as writing 22 books explaining how the food we eat and the liquids we drink have a direct effect on our health. During that time, it has been an honour to work with many great pioneers of what Linus Pauling called 'orthomolecular medicine', which simply translates as 'giving the body the right molecules'. He believed that 'optimum nutrition is the medicine of tomorrow', and he was right.

Since the foundation of ION, great advances have been made, with new research being published almost daily, proving the inextricable linking of health, disease and nutrition. What those of us at the cutting edge of this new science have proven, day after day, in our clinics and with our research, is now finally being heralded by many as 'the truth', as an abundance of research studies report on the restorative power of nutrients. For many years nutritional therapists have been treating people who are unwell – whether vertically ill (upright but not feeling great) or horizontally ill (debilitated). These people have often consulted the therapists as a last resort, and we have seen clients restored to health and well-being beyond their wildest dreams.

You, too, can have optimum health – and there's no better way to kick-start it than with my 9-Day Liver Detox! Many of us recognise that some foods and drinks instantly make us feel good, and we may also know that there are other foods whose beneficial effects we feel the day after – perhaps making us feel more energised or refreshed. So we may already have an idea of what good nutrition does for us. Although many people have the mistaken idea that nutritionists are 'born' virtuous and healthy, the truth is that most of us, just like you, have discovered optimum nutrition as the only sustainable solution for our own health problems or to create that feeling of well-being.

# Why a liver detox?

This detox programme concentrates on the liver, so you may be wondering why the liver is such an important organ in the body. In fact the liver is the greatest multi-tasking organ, and as a result its function – or dysfunction – has an incredibly important impact on our health; the following are the liver's main functions:

**Breaking down and eliminating toxins.** The liver is the organ of detoxification. When it is not working properly, toxins from both inside and outside the body remain in the system and can cause your immune system to treat them as if they were invading organisms. This can lead to many health problems including inflammation, increased likelihood of infections, and food allergies and sensitivities.

**Breaking down and eliminating excess hormones.** When this function is not working optimally, all kinds of hormonal imbalances can occur, promoting health problems from pre-menstrual syndrome (PMS) to acne.

**Balancing blood sugar.** When our blood-sugar levels are high (for example, just after consuming sugary foods and drinks), the hormone insulin triggers the liver to store the excess as glycogen. When blood-sugar levels fall, the liver releases glycogen to be turned into glucose. If the liver fails in this task, the result is chronic fatigue, sugar cravings, weight gain and, ultimately, diabetes.

**Producing bile.** This vital substance helps digestion, by breaking down fat and removing excess cholesterol. Without it, cholesterol levels rise and many digestive disorders can result, including bloating, irritable bowel syndrome (IBS), nausea, food allergies and the malabsorption of nutrients, especially the fat-soluble vitamins A, D, E and K.

**Storing nutrients.** The liver stores many essential vitamins and minerals, including iron, copper, vitamins A, $B_{12}$, D, E and K.

In fact, just about any allergic, inflammatory or metabolic disorder may involve or create impaired liver function, increasing inflammation in the body resulting in eczema, asthma, chronic fatigue, chronic infections, inflammatory bowel disorders, multiple sclerosis and rheumatoid arthritis, to name but a few, which in turn affect liver function.

Because the liver struggles valiantly on, working hard, it can be some time before serious symptoms of dysfunction appear. However, you may find that you are feeling tired and sluggish – this is a possible sign that your liver may benefit from a detox. You can check whether a detox would be beneficial for you by completing my questionnaire on page 12.

# Are liver detoxes safe?

In the old days of total fasts, where you drank only water, naturopaths used to talk about the 'healing crisis' where you felt worse before you felt better. But often this was really just a crisis! For safety, our bodies store toxins in our adipose tissue (fat stores). When we lose weight rapidly, those toxins are released, and the liver – as an organ of detoxification – has to deal with them. The idea of a liver detox is to support and take the load off the organ by providing the nutrients it needs – not to give it even more work to do!

My 9-Day Liver Detox is built on nothing but sound nutritional principles. It aims to support your liver's ability to do its job detoxing your body by removing anti-nutrients – in other words, toxins – from the diet and replacing them with the very nutrients it needs for optimum efficiency. You will not be starving yourself at any point; our 9-Day Menu Plan is carefully crafted, consisting of tasty, nutritious and filling recipes so that you will never go hungry. Instead, you will be taking in a large quantity of the nutrients that are directly beneficial to your liver and which will actively support its detoxification function. It can then do its job of safely removing toxins from your fat stores and processing them appropriately without any ill effects.

Of course, if you are addicted to caffeine and go cold-turkey while you follow the detox, you may feel worse for a couple of days, but soon you'll have more energy than ever before. You may get temporary withdrawal symptoms when you stop eating foods that you are intolerant to, but taking the recommended supplements really helps to minimise them. What you will be including in your diet will support not only your liver but the rest of your body, including your brain.

# What benefits will I experience?

If you follow the steps in my 9-Day Liver Detox carefully, you should enjoy:

- Increased energy and vitality
- Clearer skin
- Freedom from digestive complaints
- Regular bowel movements
- Fresh breath
- Clearer sinuses
- Fewer infections
- Brighter eyes
- Sharper mind

You may even want to stay on the plan for longer, for even more noticeable benefits.

# Practising what we preach

Fiona McDonald Joyce, who has provided all the wonderful recipes for this book, is a qualified ION nutritional therapist and cookery consultant. Her speciality is making what's good for you taste great. In the run up to her wedding and while she was devising these recipes, she followed my 9-Day Liver Detox herself to sort out some skin problems. She is happy to report great results – she looked absolutely radiant on her wedding day!

I am passionate about the healing power of my 9-Day Liver Detox and it was just what I needed recently, having just completed a gruelling lecture tour abroad, followed by a house move and combined with some overindulgence over Easter. Within just two days I felt completely recharged and back to tip-top health. It's amazing how good you can feel in such a short space of time.

Throughout this book you will read lots more first-hand experiences of what it is like to cut out favourite foods and the importance of having appetising recipes when you are craving 'off-limits' foods. You'll discover many recipes that are appetising, interesting and positively packed with nutrients that will become staples in your repertoire long after the nine days, making my 9-Day Liver Detox a highly doable and actually an enjoyable experience.

The detox programme will give you foods that superboost your liver's ability to detoxify, plus liver-friendly supplements, so that you will start to feel better almost immediately. One sceptical journalist, Zoe Strimpel from the *Daily Telegraph*, 'test-drove' the detox only, without the supplements, *for just one day* and said, 'I must admit, I felt clear-headed and wholesome.'

Let's face it – change is difficult. But the fear is usually of leaving the known – of breaking your unconscious food habits and doing something different. Once you start eating new foods that taste great and fill you up, it is remarkably easy. Here's how the book is arranged:

- Chapters 1, 2 and 3 explain exactly how your liver detoxifies, the five habits to break and the five habits to make, and the reasons behind them, to make your detox successful.

- Chapter 4, Test Your Detox Potential – Before and After, helps you identify, and quantify, your need to detox, both with questionnaires and a simple urine test that measures your detox potential.

- Chapter 5, Start Detoxing Now!, tells you exactly what you need to do.

- Chapter 6, Your 9-Day Liver-detox Recipes, gives you the exact daily menus and recipes so that you can follow the detox to the letter if you wish, or adapt it as you like according to your tastes.

- Chapter 7, Your Liver Detox for Life, explains how to reintroduce foods after the nine-day programme, and how to learn what suits you in the process, and then to incorporate my detox principles into your daily life.

Overall, I expect you to enjoy the experience and love the results when you reach the end. It does take courage and commitment to say no to the pub and to the millions of high-street temptations, even for a week, but as you progress on the detox you will feel so many benefits that they will spur you on to continue. I wish you well and, as the old Chinese proverb says, 'Perseverance furthers'.

Wishing you the best of health,

*Patrick and Fiona*

# CHAPTER **ONE**

# Why Detox?

Some people say that all you need to do to detox your body is to drink water and cut back on the booze, so is detoxifying a myth and detox diets just a fad? In this chapter I will explain how toxins can build up in your body and create health problems and how detoxing using supplements to assist the process can return you to a feeling of good health.

In this book you will learn that your body expends as much effort detoxifying toxins as it does building new cells, but your ability to detoxify is finite. Each of us is unique, both in which toxins we react to and in our ability to clear them from our body. When your body is detoxifying efficiently the immediate effect is that you feel better, but efficient detoxification also has the potential to extend your healthy life, so understanding how detoxification works is an essential step towards improving your overall health. There are two sides to detoxifying: the first is to reduce the toxins your body is exposed to and the second is to improve your body's ability to detoxify. There are three main areas in your body where this takes place: your digestive tract, your liver and your immune system – and this means that your whole body is involved in the process.

My 9-Day Liver Detox is not like one of the faddy detox diets that you may have tried or read about. All of its principles are based on scientific fact (and for those who want to check them I've not only listed all the references to the studies in the book but you can also click on www.patrickholford.com/detoxreferences and go straight to many of them). This is science – not science fiction.

The reason why detox diets are so popular is that many people – probably including yourself – are well aware that you feel under par after a period of excess; this might be after too much sugar, caffeine, alcohol, fried food, overeating, active or passive smoking, pollution or drugs. But you may also feel that your body has been affected by certain environments – perhaps 'mouldy' places or places that involve chemical exposure, for example – or after you have eaten certain foods. These are all examples of substances the body has to work hard to detoxify. Exactly how the body does this is the key to understanding how to boost your detox potential and feel better faster.

## Our health now

Most of us are vertically ill – that is, we are upright but don't feel great. At these times, the balance between our intake of toxins and our ability to detoxify is not at its best. Some of us become horizontally ill, and keel over when our intake of toxins exceeds our body's capacity to detoxify. Excess alcohol is an example of such a situation. When the liver's capacity to detoxify the alcohol you are consuming is exceeded, your brain becomes intoxicated and you become unable to stay conscious. Another example is the painkiller paracetamol. When your liver is unable to detoxify the drug any longer you'll collapse and, provided you make it to the hospital in time, you'll be pumped full of a detoxifying nutrient called glutathione to increase your liver's detoxing potential – and your liver will be back on track. Many old people die when their liver's ever-decreasing ability to detoxify is overloaded.

Right now you are probably somewhere between these extremes of optimal and minimal detox potential. If you have the time and money, you can actually test your liver's ability to detoxify (more on this in Chapter 4). For now, though, you can get an instant impression of your detox potential by completing the questionnaire below, which lists the symptoms associated with a reduced detox potential. Score yourself now and then retake the questionnaire and compare the score after completing my 9-Day Liver Detox.

## QUESTIONNAIRE check your detox potential

Complete this questionnaire to discover whether you need to improve your detoxification potential:

1. Do you often suffer from headaches or migraine? ☐

2. Do you sometimes have watery or itchy eyes, or swollen, red or sticky eyelids? ☐

3. Do you have dark circles under your eyes? ☐

4. Do you sometimes have itchy ears, earache, ear infections, drainage from the ears or ringing in the ears? ☐

5. Do you often suffer from excessive mucus, a stuffy nose or sinus problems? ☐

6. Do you suffer from acne, skin rashes or hives? ☐

7. Do you sweat a lot and have a strong body odour? ☐

8. Do you sometimes have joint or muscle aches or pains? ☐

9. Do you have a sluggish metabolism and find it hard to lose weight, or are you underweight and find it hard to gain weight? ☐

10. Do you often suffer from frequent or urgent urination? ☐

11. Do you suffer from nausea or vomiting? ☐

12. Do you often have a bitter taste in your mouth or a furry tongue? ☐

13. Do you have a strong reaction to alcohol? ☐

**14.** Do you suffer from bloating?

**15.** Does coffee leave you feel jittery or unwell?

Total

## Score

**7 or more** If you answer yes to seven or more questions you need to improve your detox potential.

**4–7** If you answer yes to between four and seven questions you are beginning to show signs of poor detoxification and need to improve your detox potential.

**Fewer than 4** If you answer yes to fewer than four questions, you are unlikely to have a problem with detoxification.

# Anyone can benefit from the detox

If you have discovered that you are experiencing several of the symptoms listed above you will benefit the most from my 9-Day Liver Detox, but the principles of the diet are also good for anybody who just wants to feel great. People who have followed the programme often report that they now experience:

- Better energy
- A clearer mind
- Waking up alert and refreshed
- No more bloating
- A clear nose – not blocked up
- No more bags or dark circles under the eyes
- Easier weight loss
- Better digestion

- Better and more 'alive' skin

- No more water retention

- No more PMT

- Fewer aches and pains

- No more infections

To help you continue to enjoy better health, once you have completed the detox, which requires you to remove foods that can cause intolerances, I'll explain how to reintroduce those potentially offending foods and drinks to help you define your perfect diet for daily living.

## How toxic are you?

Our bodies are permanently under assault from toxins. There are those outside our bodies that come from our environment, there are those that our own bodies make, and, of course, there are those toxins that we put into our bodies ourselves.

The liver is the clearing house for all these toxins. When it cannot process (detoxify) toxins fast enough because of overload, the toxins have to be stored in the body to be dealt with later. Guess where they are stored? In the fat cells. So we put on weight and inches not only because of our unhealthy eating habits but also to accommodate all these unprocessed toxins. When the liver is ready to cope with these additional toxins, they are released from the fat cells for processing and are transported via the lymphatic system (the transport system for fat molecules), the kidneys and the blood. This makes it easier for your body to shed the weight and inches through healthy eating and exercise, because now the fat cells are not clinging on to the toxins in an attempt to protect your body from their effects.

When these toxins stay in the body, the whole system literally becomes intoxicated. Many hundreds of different symptoms and health problems can result from a liver that is having difficulty coping with excess toxins, including the ones illustrated in the diagram on the opposite page.

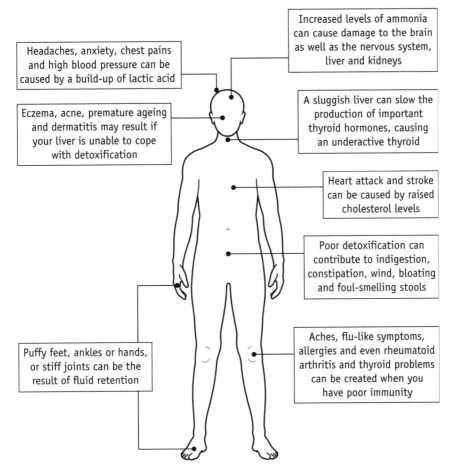

Increased levels of ammonia can cause damage to the brain as well as the nervous system, liver and kidneys

Headaches, anxiety, chest pains and high blood pressure can be caused by a build-up of lactic acid

A sluggish liver can slow the production of important thyroid hormones, causing an underactive thyroid

Eczema, acne, premature ageing and dermatitis may result if your liver is unable to cope with detoxification

Heart attack and stroke can be caused by raised cholesterol levels

Poor detoxification can contribute to indigestion, constipation, wind, bloating and foul-smelling stools

Puffy feet, ankles or hands, or stiff joints can be the result of fluid retention

Aches, flu-like symptoms, allergies and even rheumatoid arthritis and thyroid problems can be created when you have poor immunity

**Problems that can result from a faulty liver**

## Skin complaints

Like the liver, the skin is also an organ of detoxification. When your liver isn't working optimally, your skin will try to eliminate toxins. This can cause a variety of unpleasant side effects such as premature ageing, acne, eczema and dermatitis.

## Poor digestion

Without bile, which is produced in the liver and stored in the gall bladder, you cannot digest fat. If fats are not being 'emulsified' – that is, made water soluble – they will pass into the large intestine for elimination. Bile also stimulates peristalsis, which is the muscular movement of the digestive tract that propels food along it. A sluggish bowel results in constipation; when, finally, there is a bowel movement, the stool will contain greasy, undigested fat and will smell foul!

Fats are an important part of a healthy diet, and contained in them are the fat-soluble vitamins A, D, E and K, which are essential for health. Signs of their deficiency include:

- Susceptibility to colds and infections
- Feeling of being 'run down' and tired
- Skin complaints
- Poor hair condition
- Bleeding gums
- Stress-related disorders
- Poor night vision
- Burning sensation in the mouth and throat
- Insomnia
- Lack of sex drive
- Exhaustion after light exercise
- Easy bruising
- Slow wound healing
- Varicose veins
- Poor skin elasticity
- Loss of muscle tone
- Infertility

Other unpleasant side effects of poor digestion include:

- Indigestion
- Bad breath

- Nausea

- Bloating

- Constipation and diarrhoea

- Irritable bowel syndrome

- Weight gain

## Poor immunity

The liver contains many immune cells that clean up debris from the blood as it travels through the liver for cleaning. When the liver is compromised and foreign particles flow back into the bloodstream, the immune system launches an attack. As result, you are more likely to suffer from hard-to-shift infections, flu-like symptoms, allergies and even possibly autoimmune diseases like rheumatoid arthritis and thyroid problems.

## Raised cholesterol

The liver produces HDLs – high-density lipoproteins known as 'good cholesterol'. They have an important job to do, travelling around the body collecting any excess cholesterol and transporting it out of the arteries and back to the liver. From there it is taken away in bile and excreted in the stool. With poor bile flow, the cholesterol accumulates and your risk for a heart attack or stroke increases. It can also be reabsorbed in the gut unless you have consumed enough fibre.

## Fluid retention

Almost all the proteins found in the blood are made in the liver. Among their many tasks, blood proteins, particularly albumin, help to maintain correct fluid balance. If you are experiencing fluid retention (such as unexplained weight gain, puffy feet, ankles or hands, or stiff joints) it may mean that your liver is not processing proteins efficiently.

## Ammonia poisoning

You may be familiar with the sharp, penetrating smell of ammonia. It's so strong that one waft of 'smelling salts' under the nostrils can bring someone out of a faint. However, more than just a sniff of this toxic, reactive and corrosive gas can cause serious illness or even be fatal.

All proteins are made up of amino acids and, when they are broken down, they release ammonia. This then travels to the liver for removal from the blood and conversion into urea, which is excreted in the urine. Ammonia is also released in the kidneys, but what isn't excreted in urine travels back to the liver. If the liver is overworked, ammonia conversion into urea slows down, leaving an 'ammonia pool', which has to be released into the blood. You might think you would know if you had an ammonia overload. Of course, if it were that bad you would be very ill indeed, but just a slight excess in circulating ammonia can cause damage to the brain, nervous system, liver and kidneys.

## Lactic acid poisoning

Lactic acid is a toxin released from our cells when energy production is impaired because the liver has not been able to store enough B vitamins due to overload. Excess lactic acid is very common in chronic fatigue and causes aching muscles after only a small amount of exertion. A build-up of lactic acid can also cause panic attacks, anxiety, headaches, brain fog, chest pains and soaring blood-pressure levels.

I hope that this brief tour around liver function has convinced you that this vital organ is worth looking after. You can start by giving it a holiday when you embark on my 9-Day Liver Detox.

# The two sides of the detox coin

'What is food to one man is bitter poison to others,' said Lucretius (99–55 BC), the Roman healer and philosopher, some 2,000 years ago. But there are common substances that we all consume that promote our health and well-being, whereas there are others that we know adversely affect our health. We can call the good guys nutrients and the bad guys toxins – or anti-nutrients, if you prefer.

The two sides of detoxification are to decrease the toxins, which your body struggles to remove, and to increase the nutrients, which your body needs both to stay well and to improve your ability to detoxify the anti-nutrients.

# What are toxins?

The single greatest toxin the body has to detoxify every second of every day is the product of oxidation (oxidants). Oxidants can damage the cells in our bodies if they are allowed to remain, just the same way that rust will damage iron if it is allowed to form.

Many of these oxidants originate within the body as a normal process of energy creation in the cells, as fats and glucose are 'burned' with oxygen. That's how we stay alive, so oxidation is not intrinsically bad. It's the products of oxidation that can cause harm if not dealt with appropriately. But there are other oxidants that come to us from outside, either in our food or the air we breathe. For example, eating burned or fried food, breathing in exhaust fumes or smoking cigarettes (including other people's) exposes us to oxidants. In fact, one single puff of a cigarette contains a trillion oxidants. These oxidants, regardless of source, are known as 'free radicals', and they are highly reactive chemicals, which can cause a lot of damage to our cells if they are not neutralised properly. Fortunately, there are ways of neutralising the free radicals (this is covered in Chapter 3).

We all suffer from the effects of oxidants, but other toxins don't affect each of us in the same way. Finding out what is toxic for you is half the battle towards improved health and well-being. We can call whatever makes you feel worse an 'intolerance'. In some cases it might be a substance that just overloads your detox potential, such as alcohol or caffeine (found in coffee and other caffeinated drinks). For some people, the tiniest amount of alcohol or caffeine makes them feel unwell, whereas others can tolerate large amounts. In any case, we all benefit from minimal exposure to substances that the liver has to detoxify, whether they come from external or internal sources, including:

- **Caffeine and alcohol** (see Chapter 2).

- **High-meat diets** (and particularly burned meat; for example, barbecued meat, see Chapter 2). Meat can alter the body's acid balance for the worse and cause inflammation.

- **Saturated and damaged fats.** These can damage cell membranes and are also a source of inflammation (damaged fats are discussed in Chapter 2).

- **Salt,** which is a stomach irritant, linked to gastric cancer, and which also raises blood pressure.

- **Processed foods** high in chemical flavour enhancers, such as tartrazine and MSG, or preservatives such as benzoates.

- **Recreational and medicinal drugs.** These place an enormous load on the liver, especially painkillers; the average person in Britain takes over 300 of them in a year!

- **Environmental pollutants,** which include cigarette smoke, exhaust fumes, paint fumes, pesticides and fertilisers found in non-organic foods, heavy metals from dental materials and non-organic foods.

It's best to avoid any of the above that you can and to minimise your exposure to the remainder.

In other cases your intolerance will be an actual allergy, which means that your immune system 'attacks' the substance in question, be it grass pollen, moulds, yeast, wheat or milk. Allergies come in different shapes and sizes, from full-blown immediate allergies (usually based on a kind of antibody called IgE attacking the offending item) causing immediate reactions, to 'hidden' or delayed allergies (based on IgG antibodies). Many people have these without even knowing it, but feel worse as a result. My 9-Day Liver Detox eliminates the most common food allergens and shows you how to reintroduce foods to narrow down those that rob you of vitality. Of course, the best way to find out whether you have any allergies is to have a food intolerance test (see Resources).

## How your liver detoxifies

If eating the right food is one side of the coin, detoxification is the other. From a chemical perspective, much of what goes on in the body involves substances being broken down, built up and turned from one thing into another. A good 80 per cent of this work in the body involves detoxifying potentially harmful substances. Much of this work is done by the liver, which represents a clearing house able to recognise millions of potentially harmful chemicals and transform them into something harmless or prepare them for elimination. This often means turning a fat-based toxin into something water-soluble that can be eliminated in the urine. The liver is the chemical brain of the body: recycling, regenerating and detoxifying in order to maintain your health.

The external toxins, or exo-toxins, listed on page 20 represent just a small part of what the liver has to deal with; many toxins are made within the body from otherwise harmless molecules. Every breath and every action can generate toxins. So, too, can and do the bacteria and yeasts that live inside us. These internally created toxins, or endo-toxins, have to be disarmed and eliminated in just the same way that exo-toxins do. If they are not eliminated, the body becomes irritated and inflamed. Antibodies formed to protect us against the harmful effect of potential toxins often trigger an autoimmune response, so our body actually starts fighting itself. If toxins can't be broken down they are stored in the liver and in fat.

So, whether a substance is bad for you depends as much on your ability to detoxify it as on its inherent toxic properties. If your ability to detoxify is overloaded, you may have more toxins in your system and, on top of that, other key functions in the liver may be impaired; for example, the liver's ability to activate vitamins and minerals, which it needs to process to become effective, or its ability to burn fat for energy.

My 9-Day Liver Detox gives your liver a holiday as well as providing an eating plan and recommended supplements that help your liver detoxify any residual toxins. Let me explain why these foods and supplements help you detox.

# Liver detoxification is a two-step dance

The ability of the liver to detoxify has two distinct phases. You can think of Phase 1 as the preparation phase, where toxins are acted on by a series of enzymes (called P450). This phase converts toxins into a form that can be disarmed. Often, however, this process itself can produce unwanted by-products or 'reactive intermediates' such as free radicals that act as toxins. To avoid this Phase-1 side effect there is a whole series of nutrients, particularly antioxidants, that you need to support your liver.

## Detox nutrients – the Phase-1 heroes

The first phase of liver detoxification (the grey area above the line in the illustration opposite), which involves the P450 family of enzymes, mainly depends on having a great supply of antioxidant nutrients. These include:

**Glutathione** and/or **N-acetyl cysteine**[1] – found in onions and garlic

**Coenzyme Q10**[2] – found in oily fish, spinach, raw seeds and nuts

**Vitamin C**[3] – found in broccoli, peppers, citrus fruit and berries

**Vitamin E**[4] – found in raw seeds, nuts and fish

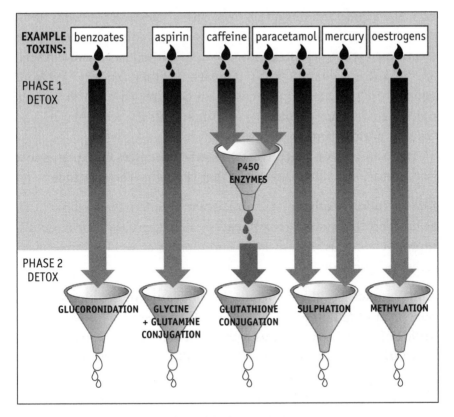

**How the liver detoxifies**

**Selenium**[5] – found in raw seeds, nuts and fish

**Beta-carotene**[6] – found in carrots, peaches, watermelon, sweet potato and butternut squash

These antioxidants are team players. You need all of them for your detox potential to be optimum. You may have seen newspaper headlines claiming that some recent research shows that antioxidants confer no benefits. This is because antioxidants are tested alone, whereas in fact they work best in synergy with other antioxidants. For example, in one study beta-carotene given on its own to smokers had slightly increased their risk of cancer, but reduced the risk if given in combination with other antioxidants.[7] Vitamin E generally reduces your risk of heart disease as part of a multivitamin, but not if you take a large amount on its own with cholesterol-lowering statin drugs.[8] This is because cholesterol-lowering statin drugs knock out coenzyme Q10 (CoQ10), another natural antioxidant, which is vital for 'reloading' vitamin E to detoxify another oxidant. Without enough CoQ10 vitamin E becomes an oxidant – a toxin in its own right. (See diagram on page 63 – Antioxidants are team players – to see how antioxidants work together.)

There are also various phytonutrients (substances from plants that have nutritional value) and herbs that can help. These include:

**DIM (Di-IndolylMethane)** – a substance in cruciferous vegetables such as broccoli that helps detoxify excess oestrogens and hormone disrupting chemicals such as PCBs and dioxins as well as some herbicides and pesticides.[9]

**Bioflavonoids**[10] – these include **anthocyanidins** in blueberries[11], **quercetin** in red onions[12], **polyphenols** in green tea[13] and the herb **Milk Thistle**, which contains a powerful detoxifying nutrient called **silymarin** that protects liver cells from all kinds of toxins.[14]

Foods rich in these nutrients are included in my 9-Day Liver Detox recipes, as well in the detox supplements I recommend (see page 104).

At Phase 2 these reactive intermediates are rendered non-toxic. This happens by enzymes linking the toxin to another molecule that makes it more water-soluble and less toxic. This process is often called 'conjugation' where the toxin is 'married' to a key detoxifying nutrient. For example, the diagram opposite shows you how your body detoxifies paracetamol, aspirin and caffeine. (You'll see on page 72 how a simple urine test that involves taking a measured amount of caffeine, paracetamol and aspirin can determine your liver's detox capacity.)

The body processes toxins in the liver using different chemical pathways. Shown here are examples of what the liver does with caffeine, paracetamol (acetaminophen) or aspirin. These different pathways (for example, glutathione conjugation or sulphation), need different nutrients to work properly.

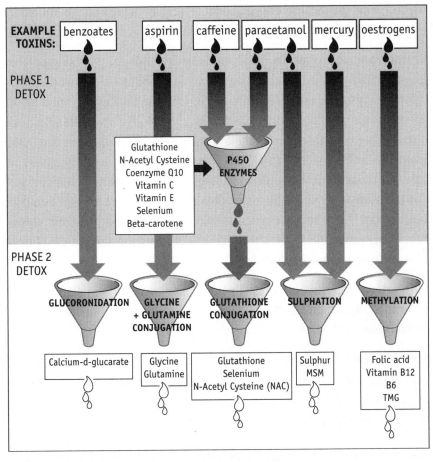

**The key detox nutrients your liver needs**

## Detox nutrients – the Phase-2 heroes

In Phase 2 the liver detoxifies substances by attaching things on to them so that they are ready to be eliminated from the body in the process called conjugation described above. There are five main ways in which the liver detoxifies:

**Glucoronidation** is possibly the most important detox pathway of all, dependent on calcium-d-glucarate, which is found in apples, Brussels sprouts, broccoli, cabbage, and beansprouts.[15]

**Glycine and glutamine conjugation.** These are amino acids found in root vegetables and sprouts.

**Glutathione conjugation.** This pathway depends on a good supply of glutathione, an amino-acid complex made from three amino acids (glycine, cysteine and glutamic acid). Onions and garlic are a good source. Root vegetables are also rich in glycine. The mineral selenium also helps glutathione to work. Glutathione can be made in the body from n-acetyl cysteine (NAC), a substance that is usually given in cases of paracetamol overdose to trigger the liver into detoxifying.[16] Glutathione is recycled by anthocyanidins in berries as well as alpha lipoic acid,[17] so supplementing with both anthocyanidins (blueberries are particularly rich in these) and glutathione plus alpha lipoic acid, is much more powerful.

**Sulphation** depends on the sulphur-containing amino acids, found in onions, garlic and eggs. There's a type of sulphur you can supplement, called MSM, that helps the body detoxify.

**Methylation** is a key detoxifying process that depends on B vitamins, especially folic acid (in greens and beans), vitamin B12 (animal source only), B6, as well as tri-methyl glycine (TMG), once again found in root vegetables.

You don't need to know the chemistry but you do need to know that each of these foods, rich in key detox nutrients, are included in the 9-Day Liver Detox diet recipes and daily menus. In addition, I also recommend taking specific detox nutrients to provide additional liver support (see page 66).

# Maintaining the right balance

The final key factor in supporting the detoxification pathways is maintaining the right acid–alkaline balance in the body. The correct balance is one that is not too acid. When foods are metabolised by the body, a residue is left that can alter the body's acidity and alkalinity. Depending on the chemical composition of the metabolised foods ('ash') the food is called acid-forming or alkaline-forming. However, this is not the same as the immediate acidity of a food. Oranges, for example, are acid due to their citric acid content, but citric acid is completely metabolised and the net effect of eating an orange is to alkalise the body, so oranges are classified as alkaline-forming.

Protein is made of amino acids, and is acid-forming. Foods such as fruits and vegetables are high in potassium and magnesium. These foods, as well as seeds and nuts, are also high in calcium. They have a more alkaline effect on the body because the minerals they contain are alkaline. Your body can and does compensate, keeping the blood at the right pH; however, excessively high acid-forming diets are not good for you. Your 9-Day Liver Detox is more alkaline-forming, by virtue of including plenty of fresh fruit and vegetables in your diet. Roughly 80 per cent of our diet should come from alkaline-forming foods, and 20 per cent from acid-forming foods. The table on the following page shows which foods are which.

## Heal your digestive tract – and take a load off your liver

Whereas your liver does most of the detoxing, effectively filtering and cleansing the blood of toxic material, your digestive tract, which represents a surface area the size of a tennis court, is the gateway between the food you eat and your bloodstream. It is actually the first line of detoxification, with the gut bacteria helping to neutralise unwanted microorganisms, while the digestive enzymes help to break down food into the right pieces to enter your body.

That tennis court inside you can be healthy or unhealthy. If it is unhealthy it will become more permeable, which means that larger food particles not on the 'guest list', so to speak, will get into the bloodstream and this is called leaky gut syndrome. Whole food proteins, rather than their constituent amino acids will gatecrash into your bloodstream and your body's policemen – antibodies – will attack, forming what is known as an 'immune complex'. This is then

# Acid, neutral and alkaline foods

| High acid | Medium acid | Neutral | Medium alkaline | High alkaline |
|---|---|---|---|---|
|  | Brazil nuts |  |  | Almonds |
|  | Walnuts |  |  | Coconut |
| Edam | Cheddar cheese | Butter |  | Milk |
| Eggs | Stilton cheese | Margarine |  |  |
| Mayonnaise |  |  | Avocados | Beans |
|  |  | Coffee | Beetroot | Cabbage |
| Fish | Herrings | Tea | Carrots | Celery |
| Shellfish | Mackerel | Sugar | Potatoes | Lentils |
|  |  |  | Spinach | Lettuce |
| Bacon | Rye |  |  | Mushrooms |
| Beef | Oats |  |  | Onions |
| Chicken | Wheat |  |  | Root vegetables |
| Liver | Rice |  |  | Tomatoes |
| Lamb |  |  |  |  |
| Veal | Plums |  | Dried fruit | Apricots |
|  | Cranberries |  | Rhubarb | Apples |
|  | Olives |  |  | Bananas |
|  |  |  |  | Berries |
|  |  |  |  | Cherries |
|  |  |  |  | Figs |
|  |  |  |  | Grapefruit |
|  |  |  |  | Grapes |
|  |  |  |  | Lemons |
|  |  |  |  | Melons |
|  |  |  |  | Oranges |
|  |  |  |  | Peaches |
|  |  |  |  | Pears |
|  |  |  |  | Raspberries |
|  |  |  |  | Tangerines |
|  |  |  |  | Prunes |

Acid ←——————|——————→ Alkaline

treated by the body as a toxin and forms the basis of most food allergies and sensitivities, which have a detrimental effect on our overall health.

So, one immediate way to help detox your body is to improve the integrity of your digestive tract. You can actually test the 'intestinal permeability' of your digestive tract (a nutritional therapist can advise you) but for now I'm going to recommend something much simpler: a teaspoon of glutamine powder.

## The G factor – your gut's best friend

Although most of your body's organs are fuelled by glucose, your digestive tract is a different story. It's a vast and highly active interface between your body and the outside world, and it needs a lot of fuel to work properly day in and day out. It runs on an amino acid called glutamine – thus sparing the glucose from your food for your brain, heart and your liver.

Not only does glutamine power your gut, it heals it as well. The endothelial cells that make up the inner lining of your digestive tract replace themselves every four days and are your most critical line of defence against developing food allergies or getting infections. As your 'inner skin', your gut takes lots of hits: alcohol, nonsteroidal anti-inflammatory drug painkillers (NSAIDs) such as aspirin or ibuprofen, antibiotics, coffee and fried food are some common gastrointestinal irritants. In Japan, people taking NSAIDs for pain and inflammation are also often instructed to take 2,000mg of glutamine 30 minutes beforehand to prevent stomach bleeding and ulceration.

Many people suffer from digestive problems and possibly food allergies. My top tip (besides avoiding allergenic foods) is to take glutamine every day during your 9-Day Liver Detox, together with digestive enzymes and a probiotic supplement (see Resources). Glutamine is the preferred food of the cells lining the intestine, so I recommend one or two heaped teaspoons (that's 4,000 to 8,000mg) of glutamine powder taken last thing at night, diluted in a glass of water. This will help your gut to heal and rejuvenate.

Under normal circumstances, most of the glutamine in your food gets used up as fuel for your gastrointestinal tract. However, about 5 per cent of it is used to make glutathione, the liver's most powerful antioxidant.

Glutathione, as we saw earlier, is made from three amino acids: glycine, cysteine and glutamic acid or glutamine. Think of them as the Three Musketeers. Glutamine is found in protein foods such as beans, fish, chicken and eggs, as well as in vegetables such as cabbage, spinach, beetroot and tomatoes. Cysteine is a sulphur-containing amino acid found in onions, garlic and eggs. And glycine is found plentifully in root vegetables. By getting more of each of these amino acids, you are providing yourself with the building blocks for glutathione, which boosts your liver and protects every single cell in your body from the dangerous oxidising chemicals: free radicals.

So that's the end of your whistle-stop tour of how your body detoxifies. Now we will go on to discover the ways you can enhance your detoxification. The next two chapters give you the reasons and the ground rules behind the Six Golden Rules of your 9-Day Liver Detox – the five habits to break (explained in Chapter 2) and the five habits to make (explained in Chapter 3). These golden rules have all been taken into account in building our daily menus and recipes for you to follow.

# CHAPTER TWO

# Five Habits to Break

To get the most powerful health transformation during your 9-Day Liver Detox I am going to ask you to break five habits. These habits are the foods and drinks that most people enjoy to some extent but which will adversely effect your liver's detoxing process, as I will explain in this chapter. The five habits to break are:

**1** Wheat

**2** Milk

**3** Caffeine

**4** Alcohol

**5** Bad fats

## Wheat – our deadly bread ✕

Bread may be a staple food for you but for many it's more of a cereal killer than a staff of life. The reason is that wheat contains a protein called gluten, and specifically a type of gluten called gliadin, which is exceedingly unfriendly to your digestive tract. As I explained in Chapter 1, foods that the body cannot digest can pass through the gut wall and are recognised as toxins in the bloodstream, so it is important to avoid these to allow the liver to focus on detoxifying the toxins that are already present without introducing new ones. As your digestive system is where detoxification starts, it's important to remove bread from your diet during your nine-day detox. However, as we don't all react to wheat in the same way it may not be necessary for you to avoid wheat after the nine days is over.

Those people who are the most wheat reactive will eventually have a digestive tract that is as flat as a pancake, because all the tiny protrusions, called villi, which create the massive surface area of your insides, will be literally destroyed. This is called coeliac disease and it affects approximately one in a hundred people (although many medical textbooks wrongly say one in 4,000).[1] Far more people, and this may possibly include you, have a lesser allergy or intolerance to wheat. So, how do you know if you are one of them? There are two ways: you can take a proper allergy blood test, or you can avoid wheat for nine days and see how you feel. If you follow this second course and find that you feel much better at the end of nine days, but worse when you reintroduce it, I recommend you have a blood test (see Resources for more details on allergy tests).

## The common symptoms of gluten allergy

If you are suffering from any of these conditions this may point to a gluten allergy:

- Sniffling and snuffling, and sinus problems
- Fatigue and chronic fatigue syndrome
- Mouth ulcers
- Anaemia
- Diarrhoea/constipation
- Abdominal bloating
- Crohn's disease or diverticulitis

- Depression

- Poor concentration and brain 'fog'

## The problem protein – gluten

As you need to avoid allergens during your detox, a little background about one of the most common ones may be helpful in understanding why wheat can be such a problem. Gluten is the key protein in wheat, but it's also found in rye, barley and oats. In fact, gluten is a name for a family of proteins found in grains. The principal type of gluten, called gliadin,[2] is found in wheat, along with glutenin, but rye and barley also contain chemically similar types of gluten (hirudin and secalin respectively), so a person who is wheat sensitive is also likely to react to barley and rye. Oats are quite different, however, because the type of gluten in oats bears no resemblance to gliadin. Approximately 80 per cent of people diagnosed with coeliac disease don't react to oats.[3]

About one in three people tested for IgG food allergy (see Chapter 1) will react to wheat. Of these, 90 per cent will react to gliadin, whereas 15 per cent will react to barley and 2 per cent will react to rye. Even fewer react to oats. Most people's immune systems react to gliadin when it gets into the bloodstream – and that may mean that you are affected. So this is why it's important to avoid wheat, as it may be recognised as a toxin in your system, as I will explain below. But first, at little about its history.

### How it all began

When it comes to eating grains, this is a relatively new food for the human race. Humankind started eating gluten grains, at the earliest, 10,000 years ago. If the history of humankind was condensed into 24 hours, we would have been eating gluten grains for, at most, six minutes. Some cultures started eating wheat only in the last 100 years – or the last two seconds. Thanks to advances in DNA research we now know that we humans shrank in height when we shifted to a grain-eating peasant diet. Our hunter–gatherer ancestors, living on meat, fish and seafood, vegetables, fruit, nuts and seeds were 13–15cm (5–6in) taller, and had 11 per cent larger brains.

All this history is encoded in your genes, and recently it has been discovered that gluten-allergic people have a genetic 'tag' called DQ2 and DQ8, which has also been revealed to be increasingly common in societies that introduced grains late, including the north-west of Europe, and especially western Ireland, and Scandinavia, where grain growing isn't easy and consequently people's bodies have not adapted over the millennia to accept gluten grains.[4]

## Why you might be sensitive to wheat

What this research is showing is that as many as one in three people in Britain may be allergic to gluten. Research shows that at least 15 per cent of wheat eaters do have gliadin in their blood.[5] Of course, if you don't eat wheat very often, and have impeccable digestion and a super-healthy digestive tract that stops any undesirables getting through, no gliadin is going to get into your bloodstream. But many of us who don't digest so well can retain gliadorphins in the blood, which are wheat-based opioids that can actually make you crave wheat products, but which we are actually allergic to according to the research of Dr Paul Shattock at Sunderland University.[6]

## How it affects the detox

The reason for avoiding wheat (and preferably all gluten grains) is that if you are sensitive to them, the immune system will treat particles of wheat as a toxic invader and send antibodies to bind themselves to them, forming what is called an 'immune complex'. Once that happens, the liver is tied up detoxifying the immune complex and is not dealing with your other toxins. Given that gliadin irritates just about anyone's gut if you have enough of it, I recommend you strictly avoid all wheat, rye and barley products, but not oats, for nine days to give your digestive system a break.

## Gliadin grains to avoid

During your detox avoid bread, cakes, biscuits, cereals or pasta made from any of these gluten grains:

Wheat

Spelt

Rye

Barley

Kamut (a new cereal that is an ancient relative of modern durum wheat, but is higher in lipids, amino acids, vitamins and minerals than wheat)

Triticale (a man-made hybrid of rye and wheat)

## Non-gliadin grains that you can enjoy

Instead, you can have bread, pasta, cereals and other foods made from these:

Oats

Amaranth (a South American gluten-free pseudograin – or false grain because it comes from a broad-leaf plant and not a grass. It is high in protein, fibre and some of the key dietary minerals)

Buckwheat

Corn

Gram (ground chickpea flour)

Maize

Millet

Quinoa

Rice

For example, you can have rice or corn-based cereals, oatcakes, gram chapattis, buckwheat pancakes, chickpea pasta, rice or buckwheat noodles, rice or quinoa with your main meal. These may be new foods for you so we're giving you loads of easy gliadin-free recipes to choose from.

# Milk – it's a four-letter word ⊗

If I were still breastfeeding at the age of 30 – from another species of animal – wouldn't you consider that rather strange? That is actually what we all do by drinking milk. Put that way it may not be so surprising that our immune systems often react against milk, as if it were an alien substance not on the body's 'guest list', and have difficulty digesting it. So, as we want to aid our digestion rather than add to its load during the detox, milk is out during your 9-Day Liver Detox.

## What's wrong with cow's milk?

Cow's milk is the most common food allergy, whichever way you look at it. A classic IgE-based allergy to milk is the most common food allergy, and so too is hidden or delayed IgG food allergy to milk.

Logically, its status as a gut irritant and an allergen isn't surprising, since it is a highly specific food, containing all kinds of hormones designed for the first few months of a calf's life. Like wheat, it's also a relatively recent addition to the human diet. Our ancestors, after all, weren't milking buffaloes. Once we have been weaned as children, approximately 75 per cent of people (25 per cent of people of Caucasian origin and 80 per cent of Asian, Native American or African origin) stop producing lactase, the enzyme that's needed to digest milk sugar, lactose. Lactase deficiency, or lactose intolerance, leads to significant diarrhoea, bloating, cramping and excess gas – all of which can increase gut permeability and, as a result, it places a greater detox load on the liver. Between 18 months and four years after birth, most Asian, Hispanic, Afro-American, Native American and Caucasians of southern European descent gradually lose lactase – one of many clues that the human body isn't designed to drink cow's milk, at least beyond early childhood.[7]

# How will milk affect the detox?

It's not the lactose – the sugar in milk – that causes milk allergy, however. It's the protein. In other words, you can be either lactose intolerant, or milk protein allergic, or both; that is, often lactose intolerance and milk allergy occur together. I recommend avoiding milk for the same reason as wheat: if you are sensitive to milk protein, the immune system will treat it as a toxic invader and antibodies will attach to it in something called an 'immune complex'. Once that happens, the liver is tied up detoxifying the immune complex and is not dealing with your other toxins. As we have seen in Chapter 1, in order for the detox to work effectively we must reduce the toxins we are eating or drinking wherever possible to allow the liver to concentrate on those toxins that are already present in our body. In addition, non-organic milk can contain traces of the hormones and antibiotics normally fed to cattle, and the pesticide and fertiliser residues from their fodder, which also have to be detoxified in the liver.

Of course, most of us have been brainwashed since childhood by the milk marketeers into believing that milk is not only a necessary food but also almost a wonder food. With that knowledge it might seem surprising that half the world, for example most of China and Africa, can survive, let alone thrive, without it. Milk is a reasonably good source of calcium, among other nutrients, but drinking milk certainly isn't the only way, or necessarily the best way, to achieve optimal nutrition. On top of that, the more you have, the greater your risk of a wide range of common diseases, including breast, prostate and colo-rectal cancer.[8] You'll be getting plenty of calcium on your 9-Day Liver Detox from other foods, including seeds, nuts and beans.

# Signs of an intolerance

The classic signs of milk allergy or lactose intolerance are:

Poor sleep
Asthma
Bronchitis

Chronic fatigue

Depression

Diarrhoea

Eczema

Frequent infections

Headaches/migraines

Heartburn

Hyperactivity

Indigestion

Rheumatoid arthritis

Rhinitis and sinus problems

If you have some of these symptoms, notice what happens during your 9-Day Liver Detox. If your symptoms clear up, I recommend you investigate the possibility that you have a milk allergy.

Milk is present in most cheeses, cream, yoghurt and butter, and is hidden in all kinds of food; sometimes it's called milk protein, whey (milk protein with the casein removed) or casein, which is the predominant type of protein – and is the most allergenic – in dairy products. You'll be amazed at how many foods contain milk: from bread and cereals, to packaged food and crisps.

## Milk products to avoid

Milk (including goat's or sheep's milk)

Cheese

Cream

Butter

Yoghurt

Ice cream

Probiotic drinks

Anything with milk solids

Whey (listed as casein on the label)

Instead, we'll give you delicious recipes that happen to be dairy-free.

## Milk alternatives

You can enjoy the following alternatives to dairy:

Rice, almond, quinoa or soya milk

Coconut milk, butter or cream

Soya yoghurt

Pumpkin-seed butter

Non-hydrogenated vegetable oil spreads

Cashew cream (made by blending cashews with rice milk)

Eggs

If you do find you feel much better after a period without dairy products, and worse when you reintroduce them, you'll find that there are many delicious alternatives including ice cream (try Booja Booja, for example), soya cheeses and pumpkin-seed butter.

## Caffeine – kick the habit ⊗

If the thought of giving up coffee causes a burst of hostility towards me, then the chances are you are currently addicted to caffeine. Of course, you will probably tell yourself that one cup of coffee can't harm you, that you've read all sorts of reports in the newspapers about coffee being high in antioxidants, that you don't even believe you could stop for nine days – or want to. But I'm sorry to say that all of this is simply denial that you've become somewhat dependent on your caffeine fix and can't imagine functioning without it. Caffeine is also found in tea and in drinks such as Diet Coke and Red Bull.

## How caffeine affects the detox

Now, I'm not asking you to quit caffeine for ever. Just for nine days. The reasons are simple. Firstly, the body treats caffeine as a toxin and, as we have seen above, we need to eliminate toxins from our diet while we follow the nine-day detox to give our liver a chance to cleanse the system. Secondly, I have witnessed so many people experience a tremendous gain in energy, mental clarity and improved mood just by stopping caffeine. Thirdly, blood-sugar balance is the long-term key to both energy and weight control but you'll never achieve good blood-sugar stability if you consume a lot of caffeine.

If you felt full of energy all the time, would you even want caffeinated drinks? If you do take caffeinated drinks to give you a pick-me-up, wouldn't you rather be naturally so full of energy that you don't need picking up? Think of this as a nine-day experiment.

## How does caffeine work?

By understanding how caffeine works you'll understand why it's a no-no on your 9-Day Liver Detox. The main reason you probably drink caffeinated drinks is that the caffeine content boosts your mood and energy. It does this by blocking the receptors for a brain chemical called adenosine. The body makes adrenalin (the hormone that is secreted in our body when we are under stress, in order to prepare our body for exertion – the 'flight or fight syndrome') from dopamine. We then normally break down dopamine and adrenalin to return to normal. Adenosine blocks dopamine breakdown, so the body ends up with more dopamine and therefore, more adrenalin. So with all that adrenalin, no wonder you feel more alert, motivated and stimulated! Although, of course, that extra adrenalin will make some people feel uncomfortable and jittery. The downside is that the body, unable to break down these stimulants, blocks its ears, so to speak, by shutting down receptors to dopamine and adrenalin, so you end up needing more adrenalin, and hence more caffeine. Caffeine reaches its peak concentration 30 to 60 minutes after consumption, after which it is inactivated by the liver, with only half its peak level left after four to six hours. However, during this time, the liver has to work very hard to detoxify the caffeine and is consequently not detoxifying your other toxins.

## Caffeine is dehydrating

Have you noticed how you have to go to the loo more frequently after drinking tea or coffee? This is because caffeine is a diuretic; that is, it encourages the body to get rid of its fluids. But the one thing you don't want when detoxing is to get rid of all your fluids, because then the toxins will just be reabsorbed into the body. Instead, you need lots of water – but we will come on to that in Chapter 3.

## Caffeine is addictive

Research shows that consuming as little as 100mg of caffeine a day can lead to withdrawal symptoms when you stop, including headache, fatigue, difficulty concentrating and drowsiness.[9] It's worth knowing that whereas a small cup of instant coffee may contain less than 100mg of caffeine, a large cup of 'designer' coffee can contain as much as 500mg – five times the 'addictive' dose. Even more chemicals are used in manufacturing decaffeinated coffee, and in the end it still contains traces of caffeine, although usually less than 5mg per regular cup, together with two other stimulants called theophylline and theobromine (which is the addictive substance in chocolate). It's better for you but not perfect.

The classic withdrawal effects from caffeine are tiredness, low mood, headaches, anger and irritability. Overnight withdrawal from caffeine can induce all these; however, headaches more commonly occur after a day off caffeine for regular consumers. Studies show that the energy levels of regular coffee consumers drop on withdrawal, but are usually higher after a week off coffee. However, when you follow your 9-Day Liver Detox, as well as taking the recommended supplements, you'll halve the time it takes to experience the energy gain and halve any symptoms of withdrawal.

Regular caffeine consumers are less alert on waking than non-consumers; however, they become equally alert on consuming the equivalent of a cup of coffee.[10] So, basically, coffee is highly effective at removing the withdrawal effects of coffee! Hand steadiness is considerably worse for those who consume 250mg a day – the equivalent of two reasonably strong coffees.

## Caffeine makes you more stressed and tired

At best, coffee has minor short-term mental and emotional benefits, but these are not sustained. A study published in the *American Journal of Psychiatry* observed 1,500 psychology students divided into four categories depending on their coffee intake: abstainers, low consumers (one cup or equivalent a day), moderate (one to five cups a day) and high (five or more cups a day). On psychological testing, the moderate and high consumers had higher levels of anxiety and depression than the abstainers, and the high consumers had a higher incidence of stress-related medical problems coupled with lower academic performance.[11]

In our Optimum Nutrition UK survey of 37,000 people, the more caffeinated drinks a person consumed the more tired they were. The symptoms that most correlated with increasing caffeine consumption were loss of energy, reduced libido, joint stiffness and, for women, menopausal symptoms.[12]

Coffee is also bad for your heart. Just one morning cup of coffee dramatically hardens your arteries, making blood vessels stiffer.[13] This is associated with an increased risk of heart attack and a good reason for older people, especially with high blood pressure, to lower their intake. Coffee, more than tea, is also now well known to increase homocysteine levels, one of the best predictors of heart attacks and strokes,[14] as well as a clear sign that your body treats coffee as a toxin. Drinking two cups of coffee a day significantly raises your homocysteine level, which means that the way in which your body detoxifies is reduced. Decaf (that is, caffeine-free coffee) still raises homocysteine by about 50 per cent of the increase of caffeinated coffee, so this effect is not caused by caffeine alone. It's believed to be in part due to another chemical in coffee called chlorogenic acid, which is also high in decaf coffees.

Coffee also appears to cause inflammation in the body, as shown by the presence of what are known as key inflammatory markers in the blood. A study involving over 3,000 people in Greece found that those consuming 200ml (7fl oz) of coffee – that's two cups – had between 28 and 30 per cent higher levels of each of three kinds of inflammatory marker compared to non-coffee consumers.[15] Inflammation is now recognised as the basis for many chronic degenerative diseases such as cancer, arthritis, cardiovascular disease and dementia, so it makes sense to reduce unnecessary exposure to inflammatory agents, particularly when they are also slowing down the liver. I use a simple measure of the liver's ability to clear caffeine from your system. This is a urine test that indicates how well your liver is detoxing (see page 72).

## Caffeine disrupts normal sleeping

The other big problem area for caffeine is sleep. When you go to sleep your melatonin levels increase. Melatonin is a hormone produced by the pineal gland in the brain when the evening becomes dark, and one of its important functions is to make you feel sleepy. Melatonin levels start to rise two hours before sleep, then peak somewhere between 2 am and 3 am before starting to fall, preparing us to wake up. Research conducted at Tel Aviv University found that volunteers given regular coffee, compared to decaf, slept an average of two hours less and halved the amount of melatonin produced.[16] The melatonin-depressing effects of caffeine last up to ten hours, making it wise to avoid caffeinated drinks after midday.

Another vital job for melatonin is as an antioxidant in Phase 1 detoxification (see pages 22–3 for other Phase 1 detox nutrients). So if you take in too much caffeine and suppress melatonin production, your liver can't detoxify so well. And finally, the body will naturally start to release stored toxins while you sleep, so if you are getting less sleep because of your caffeine intake, fewer stored toxins are being released from the fat cells to the liver. So you may lose out on some weight loss as well!

## Have a break

These are all the reasons why you need to quit caffeine during your 9-Day Liver Detox. However, after those nine days, for those die-hard addicts, the evidence of a harmful effect from drinking just one cup of coffee containing no more than 100mg of caffeine is weak. But during these nine days, give yourself, and your liver, a break from caffeinated drinks, coffee and strong tea.

If you drink more than one cup of coffee or tea a day, start reducing before you begin the 9-Day Liver Detox, otherwise you may find a lot of unpleasant withdrawal symptoms, such as headaches and nausea. These will pass after about 24 hours but can make the detox a very unpleasant experience for that period. So give yourself the best chance and don't give up caffeine altogether until you are already down to only one cup a day.

## Caffeine drinks to avoid

During your detox avoid the following:

Colas and diet colas

Red Bull and other caffeinated drinks

All coffee, including decaf

Regular black tea

Instead, you can have up to two weak cups of green tea if you wish, using the same tea bag. Green tea is much higher in polyphenols and antioxidants and, by using the same tea bag, the caffeine you'll be consuming is minimised. Also high in antioxidants is rooibosch (red bush) tea.

## Alternative drinks

Instead of caffeinated drinks, enjoy the following:

Green tea (no more than two weak cups, as above)
Rooibosch (red bush) tea
Red berry or rosehip teas
Lemon and ginger tea
Water
Juice (see page 148)

# Alcohol – give it a break ⊗

During the liver detox we want to avoid any foods or drinks that will add to the toxins already in our system or that will give our liver extra work. Putting aside any benefits a glass of red wine may have for heart health, there is no question that alcohol taxes both your liver and gut. The more alcohol you consume the more antioxidants you need. This is because alcohol is detoxified by the liver using a liver enzyme called alcohol dehydrogenase, but when you consume more alcohol than this enzyme can handle the liver will instead metabolise the alcohol to chloral hydrate, also known as Mickey Finn drops, which knocks you out. Normally alcohol is metabolised to acetaldehyde by an enzyme called acetyldehyde oxidase, and, from there, to harmless chemicals that can be excreted from the body. But if this enzyme is overloaded or underfunctioning you end up with too much circulating acetaldehyde. This very acidic and toxic substance leads to ketoacidosis – what we commonly refer to as a hangover: namely headache, nausea, mental and physical tiredness, and aching muscles. Acidosis occurs when the blood has become too acid, in this case through the toxic metabolites of alcohol. Acidosis is a cause of premature ageing and osteoporosis and can lead on to other disease states. It is a frequently reported finding in excess alcohol consumption.[17] The liver enzyme responsible for detoxifying alcohol depends on a good supply of antioxidant nutrients, especially vitamin C.

Yet, even before alcohol gets to the liver it has negative effects in the gut where it acts as an intestinal irritant. This increases the risk of increased intestinal permeability (see Chapter 1, Heal your digestive tract), which in turn increases the risk of allergic reactions to absorbed particles of incompletely digested food and to the ingredients within the alcoholic drink itself. For this reason, many beer and wine drinkers become allergic to yeast. About one in five people, on testing, have this sensitivity. In addition, wine drinkers may become sensitive to sulphites, which are added to grapes during the wine-making process to control their fermentation. Sulphites are also found in exhaust fumes, and the liver enzyme that detoxifies sulphites is dependent on molybdenum, a trace element that is frequently deficient in the diet. Organic, sulphite-free wines and champagne are better for you, the latter of which has the added bonus of being yeast-free.

## Alcohol can also cause cancer

As well as increasing intestinal permeability, alcohol wreaks havoc on intestinal bacteria and has been reported to convert gut bacteria into secondary metabolites, which increase the proliferation of cells in the colon, initiating cancer. Alcohol can also be absorbed directly into the mucosal cells that line the digestive tract, and converted into aldehyde, which then interferes with DNA repair and promotes tumours. There is also evidence that alcohol increases the risk of mouth, pharyngeal, laryngeal and oesophageal cancers (in other words, affecting all the way down the gastrointestinal tract from the mouth to the intestines) and primary liver cancer. It probably also increases the risk of colorectal and breast cancer.[18]

## Alcohol destroys nutrients

There is little question that alcohol acts as an 'anti-nutrient'. Whereas some forms of alcohol, such as stout or red wine, deliver a few nutrients, especially B vitamins, alcohol itself is a potent destroyer of these same nutrients. Chronic alcohol consumption leads to multiple deficiencies of nutrients, due to the alcohol destroying nutrients, as well as disturbing digestion and absorption, and it also suppresses the appetite. As well as the B vitamins, other nutrients are knocked out by alcohol, including vitamin C, magnesium and zinc. Drinking alcohol with a meal also reduces the amount of zinc and iron the body can absorb from the food.

Once you start to become drunk from alcohol you've exceeded your body's ability to detoxify. If, in addition, you already have increased gut permeability and perhaps an allergy to something in the drink, you're putting your body in for some punishment and may suffer cumulative ill effects on your health. You'll experience this as the dreaded 'hangover': nausea, headache, brain fog or stomach upset. And, in due course, your capacity for alcohol and ability to avoid hangovers will diminish. If your hangover is bad enough you'll probably take a painkiller or two. Both alcohol (and the painkillers) tie up the liver's detoxification processes when they could be spring-cleaning your body. (We can work out how well your liver is functioning by giving you a measured amount of aspirin, paracetamol and caffeine, then collecting a urine sample, see page 72.)

## Alcohol is dehydrating

In just the same way as caffeine, alcohol is a diuretic, encouraging your body to get rid of its fluids. Without sufficient fluids, your toxins will be reabsorbed into the body. So, it's important to have no diuretics while detoxing.

The above reasons are why there's no alcohol during your 9-Day Liver Detox. Once it's over I hope you will have a better functioning liver and digestive system and that you will continue to follow my 'optimum nutrition' principles. So, a glass of wine or beer once or up to three times a week is unlikely to have a negative impact upon your health. (But choose organic in preference.) If, on the odd occasion, you drink more, top up on vitamin C and other antioxidants before-hand, drink plenty of water alongside the alcohol, have a teaspoon of glutamine powder (see page 29) in water before you go to sleep, and exercise the next day. All this will help to minimise the damage.

## Alternative drinks

Instead of alcoholic drinks, enjoy the following:

- Diluted fruit juice
- Mineral water
- Tomato juice
- Fruit smoothies

# Bad fats – stay away from bad trans- and hydrogenated fats ⊗

There was a time when fats were just thought of as fuel for the body. But now we know that there are good fats and bad fats. The good fats are called omega-3 and 6 'essential' fats and we need to get them from our diet. The richest sources of essential fats are raw nuts, seeds and their oils, and oily, or carnivorous, fish such as salmon, mackerel, herring and tuna. Sardines are good, too.

The 'bad' fats are damaged fats. These are called trans-fats, which these days are much in the news; some British supermarkets are even working to banish them from their own-brand products. These damaged fats are found in deep-fried food and some foods containing hydrogenated vegetable oils. So, if you want to minimise your exposure to trans-fats, limit your intake of fried, and especially deep-fried, food, and don't buy foods containing hydrogenated fats. Check the list of ingredients in processed foods: if a food has the 'H' word in the ingredients, don't put it in your basket!

## Why are trans-fats so bad for you?

After you eat trans-fats, they can be taken directly into the brain where they disturb thinking processes by blocking the conversion of essential fats into vital brain fats such as GLA, DHA and prostaglandins. Twice as many trans-fats appear in the brains of people deficient in omega-3. So, a combined deficiency in omega-3 fats and an excess of trans-fats is bad news indeed. In a typical junk food diet, up to a quarter of fat intake can be these damaged trans-fats, found in a diet high in French fries, deep-fried food, doughnuts and other fast and convenience foods. Trans- and hydrogenated fats are difficult to digest and slow to detoxify, clogging up the liver for long periods when it could be dealing with your other toxins.

On top of this, eating fried food, especially deep-fried food, or any 'crispy' fat – be it crispy bacon or browned cheese – delivers a large quantity of oxidants that your body has to detoxify with antioxidants. Your 9-Day Liver Detox avoids all these foods.

## Is meat suitable for the diet?

Meat isn't necessarily bad news, however, as long as it's lean, organic and unburned. But most meat, especially processed meats, are high in fats; and, if the meat is burned, these become damaged fats. Many people think that white meat is better for you largely because it's lower in fat. But this really does depend on the animal and how it has been reared and fed. The average chicken in the 1970s had 9 grams of fat. Today, the average chicken is virtually obese, with 22 grams of fat. So, in this case, lean pork would be lower in fat than a fat chicken. However, my recommendation for these nine days is to avoid all meat – both red and white. We provide delicious meat-free recipes, so this is easy to do.

## Fats to avoid

During your detox avoid the following:

> All meat
> Fried fish and eggs
> Processed foods with 'hydrogenated' fats
> Processed fat spreads
> French fries and other fried vegetables

However, you do not have to avoid all fats, because those from nuts, seeds and fish contain the essential omega-3 and 6 fats that are vital for your health. Seeds and nuts from plants that are grown in a hot climate (sesame and sunflower, for example) are rich sources of omega-6 fats, whereas seeds from a cold climate (walnut, flax and pumpkin, for example) are high in omega-3 fats. But there's a particularly potent couple of omega-3 fats, called EPA and DHA, that are especially rich in coldwater fish with teeth. In other words, fish that eat fish: salmon, mackerel, herring and tuna. It's vital to have the right amount and balance of these fats, which is why they are built into your 9-Day Liver Detox. In addition, I also recommend you take a daily omega-3 and 6 supplement containing EPA and DHA (see page 66).

## Alternative foods you can enjoy

Try these health-giving foods during your detox (and beyond):

> Baked, poached or steamed oily fish
> Poached, boiled or lightly scrambled eggs
> Home-made mayonnaise
> Raw nut and seed spreads, such as tahini or pumpkin-seed butter
> Raw nuts and seeds
> Raw cold-pressed nut and seed oils – for cold use only, such as
>    salad dressings or drizzled on vegetables after cooking

Also, you can use steam-frying instead of frying to give foods a good flavour (see page 103).

# CHAPTER **THREE**

# Five Habits to Make

To be sure of maximum health at all times it's well worth forming some good habits. I'm going to ask you to adopt some during your 9-Day Liver Detox and urge you to continue with them after your detox has finished, as they will maximise your energy and well-being. The five habits to make are:

**1** Drink eight glasses of water each day

**2** Eat the big five superfoods each day

**3** Maximise your intake of anti-ageing antioxidants

**4** Take detoxifying supplements

**5** Do detoxifying exercises each day

## Drink eight glasses of water each day ✅

Drinking eight glasses of water – the equivalent of about 1.5 litres (2 ¾ pints) – makes an enormous difference to how you feel, especially your energy and mental clarity. Water helps to dilute toxins in the blood, for elimination via the kidneys, so drinking water helps your kidneys to function better. Your water intake can include caffeine-free teas and coffee alternatives. (Caffeine is a diuretic so it causes more water loss from the body.) So, this might mean having three hot drinks, your special 'detox juice' and four glasses of water a day. Half a lemon squeezed into a mug of hot water is another good option, as lemon is a great antioxidant detoxifier and helps the liver flush away its toxins into the bowel. You can also add a slice of ginger (another excellent antioxidant) as well as, or instead of the lemon, if you prefer.

However, 1.5 litres (2¾ pints) of water a day is really a minimum, because if the weather is hot, or if you exercise, you will need more water to replace the liquid you are losing as sweat.[1] Also, drinking more is generally helpful for the kidneys, because many toxins, both generated by the body and consumed, are eliminated via the kidneys. By diluting the concentration of these toxins in the blood the kidneys have an easier time – up to a point. It's also important to keep your body hydrated so that toxins are not reabsorbed into your body from the bowel. The maximum amount of liquids drunk should be equal to the amount the kidneys can reasonably excrete in 24 hours, and in adults this is about 2 litres (3½ pints) per day.[2] So, be aware that drinking more than you need, which is about 1.5–2 litres (2¾–3½ pints) a day under normal circumstances, isn't better for you and may be worse. This is because too much liquid does tax the kidneys and can lead to overhydration. Taken to the extreme this can kill you – a man died after drinking 10 litres (17½ pints) in an hour.

## What happens if you don't get enough?

Water has many roles throughout the body other than flushing the kidneys, including dissolving minerals, acting as a delivery system, a lubricant and a temperature regulator. Even very mild dehydration can lead to constipation, headaches, lethargy and mental confusion, while increasing the risk of urinary tract infections and renal stones.[3] When just 1 per cent of body fluids are lost, body temperature goes up and mental concentration becomes more difficult.

The thirst mechanism kicks in when we have lost between 1 per cent and 2 per cent of body water. However, the thirst reflex is often confused with hunger. If we ignore it or mistake it for hunger, dehydration can continue to about 3 per cent, where it seriously affects both mental and physical performance. Sports nutritionists have found that a 3 per cent loss of body water results in an 8 per cent loss in muscle strength. So, here are some tips to get you in the habit of drinking enough water:

- Drink a glass of water **when you wake up**. The blood and urine has the highest concentration of toxins in the morning, so drinking water helps you detoxify by diluting these toxins.

- Always drink **before you eat**. We often mistake thirst for hunger. So, especially if you are looking to lose weight, drink a glass of water before you reach for a snack or have a main meal.

- Drink two glasses of water **after you exercise**. Muscles get stiff when you exercise, and you also lose water through sweat. You need about 600ml (1 pint) of fluids an hour, depending on the severity of the exercise.

- **Keep water where you are**. Buy yourself an attractive 1 litre (1¾ pint) jug to keep on your desk at work. Fill it up with filtered water in the morning and drink it by the evening. Or buy 1 litre (1¾ pints) natural mineral water and drink it by the evening. Alternatively, travel with a water container; fill it up, and empty it, each day. One litre (1¾ pints) of water equals four glasses.

- **Drink filtered or natural mineral water**. Avoid any bottled water that isn't 'natural mineral water', even if it says 'spring' or 'pure'. Only spring water that comes from a pure source and has consistent mineral levels season by season, year on year, can be labelled 'natural mineral water'. What this means is that the water fell to earth, often hundreds of years ago, and has then gradually been pushed to the surface by underwater springs through deep bedrock cracks, purified and mineralised in the process. This water doesn't have any pesticide or nitrate contaminants found in the water table, and hence in tap water.

## Good water

The best water filters are available from The Fresh Water Filter Company – I have these fitted in my house (see Resources for details).

By the way, there's nothing wrong with *naturally* carbonated water. Carbon grabs hold of minerals. Naturally carbonated mineral water such as Badoit, therefore, contains carbonated minerals that are absorbed into the body. However, the carbon in artificially fizzy drinks can grab hold of minerals in the body and take them out. People who drink lots of fizzy drinks, also containing phosphoric acid, tend to have less bone density as a result. So, the best mineral water to drink is naturally carbonated, followed by still, followed by artificially carbonated. Pure distilled water, while good from the point of view of containing no impurities, also contains no minerals. Most natural water contains significant amounts of minerals – for example 60 to 100mg of calcium in 2 litres (3½ pints) of water. The best in this respect is Contrex, which contains a whopping 486mg of calcium per 1 litre (1¾ pints). There is also a magnesium-rich mineral water called Donat which contains a massive 1,000mg of magnesium in 1 litre (1¾ pints), so don't drink more than 350ml (12fl oz) (a large glass) a day. So, if you do only drink pure water, make sure you are getting all the minerals you need from your diet and supplements. Most important of all, whatever kind of water you drink, make sure you are having enough.

## Signs that you don't drink enough

Any combination of the symptoms below might help you become more in tune with your body's cries for water:[4]

- Are you prone to constipation?

- Are you often thirsty?

- Do you have joint problems?

- Do you feel tired?

- Are you having difficulty concentrating?

- Are you overheating?

- Do you have dry skin, mouth or lips?

- Do you get frequent infections?

- Do you have dry, brittle hair?

The other way to judge is the colour of your urine. If your urine is very strongly coloured then you're not drinking enough. This simple gauge is, however, complicated by the fact that riboflavin (vitamin $B_2$) makes the urine a fluorescent kind of yellow. (Riboflavin is found in mushrooms, cabbage, broccoli and mackerel and is more likely to affect the urine colour if you are also taking B vitamin supplements. This colour in urine shows that you are taking in adequate amounts of riboflavin.) However, it is different from the dark yellow of urine that is too concentrated due to lack of water and is easy to recognise once you get used to it. Ideally, your urine should be a light, straw-coloured yellow. If, however, your urine is often clear, like water, you may be drinking too much and would therefore not be taking in enough nutrients.

# Eat the big five superfoods every day ✅

Superfoods are simply foods that press all the right health buttons: they are packed with nutrients and antioxidants, and free from anything bad for you, including too much natural sugar. Since the goal of your 9-Day Liver Detox is to make sure everything you eat is packed with nutrients that support your liver's ability to detoxify, and totally free from toxins, one of the simplest ways to take a step towards this goal is to set yourself the rule of five superfood portions a day. Now, we've built this into your nine-day menu, so you don't need to do anything, but if you want to 'freewheel' or just want to know why they are included in my 9-Day Liver Detox, read on.

# 1 Seeds of life

Everything grows from a seed. For this simple reason seeds are jam-packed full of energy, protein and the nutrients necessary for plants to grow; and we grow from eating plants. All seeds are packed with minerals such as calcium, magnesium, manganese, molybdenum, zinc and selenium, all of which are essential for detoxification, but some seeds have more of one mineral than others. Pumpkin seeds are the highest in magnesium. Hot-climate seeds, such as sesame and sunflower, are high in the essential omega-6 fats that help to balance hormones and keep your skin healthy, whereas cold-climate seeds, such as flax and pumpkin, are higher in omega-3, vital for the health of your arteries, joints and brain.

These seed nutrients (especially vitamin E, magnesium, manganese, molybdenum and zinc) are especially important for the Phase 1 detoxification described on page 22. In fact zinc is essential for the Phase 1 detoxification of alcohol, so you might consider supplementing before a night out! All these minerals, with the addition of selenium, are essential for manufacturing many of the conjugation enzymes in Phase 2 detoxification. In addition, the essential fats in seeds speed up the time it takes for stools to be moved along the gut before a bowel movement, so that fewer toxins are absorbed or reabsorbed from the gut into the bloodstream.

Using a combination of these seeds provides the best all-round superfood (but please don't buy roasted seeds or you will lose much of their benefit). You need a mixture of half flax seeds, and half sesame, sunflower and pumpkin seeds. This is what I call my Essential Seed Mix (see page 109 for how to prepare this). This gives the correct balance of minerals and omega-3 and 6 essential fats, and it tastes great. Mix these seeds together and keep in an airtight container in the fridge. No light, no heat and no extra exposure to oxygen will keep them fresher for longer. Grind them as you need them in your now-redundant coffee grinder – this allows you to get the most nutrients out of the seeds. In case you are wondering, they won't make you fat. So your 9-Day Liver Detox will contain a tablespoon of this Essential Seed Mix per day.

> ### ESSENTIAL SEED MIX
>
> Have a tablespoon every day of ground seeds. Seeds are incredibly rich in essential fats, minerals, vitamin E, protein and fibre.

## 2 Go for greens

There's something special about darker green vegetables. They are packed with vitamin C, folate and chlorophyll, all of which are exceedingly good for you. To give you an example of the benefits of folate, Dr Jane Durga from Wageningen University in the Netherlands asked 818 people aged from 50 to 75 to take part in some research. Over a period of three years she gave some of the group a supplement containing 800mcg of the B vitamin folic acid a day (called folate in food) – which is what you'll receive every day on your 9-Day Liver Detox – and gave the others a dummy pill. On memory tests, the supplement users had scores comparable to people 5.5 years younger![5] As well as the benefits of folate, eating vitamin-C rich foods is linked to better skin, better energy and a substantially lower risk of cancer.[6]

Of course, these are only three of dozens of vital nutrients found in greens, but some greens are better than others. Spinach is the highest in folic acid, giving 204mcg in a cup, or a good handful, which is what you'll be having every day. Other great sources are watercress, basil and parsley. You'll be having a handful of each of these in my Super Greens Mix, giving you 800mcg a day – enough to give your memory a definite boost.

Also excellent is avocado, which you can add to the Super Greens Mix for a thicker consistency. You'll be adding the Super Greens Mix, blended, to soups, salads and other savoury foods. We'll show you how on page 122. All you need is a blender.

Watercress, parsley and basil are exceptional sources of beta-carotene (second only to carrots) and great sources of vitamin C (second only to broccoli and green peppers). All these super greens are packed full of bioflavonoids, which are special antioxidants that help your liver to detox your body. The combination is quite delicious and can be adapted to make pesto, soups, stews and salads.

> ## SUPER GREENS MIX
>
> Have a serving every day of our Super Greens Mix (see page 122 for how to prepare this) – a blend of a handful each of baby spinach leaves, watercress, parsley and basil with variations, such as sunblush tomatoes, artichoke hearts, pine nuts, pumpkin seeds and avocado.

## 3 Cruciferous vegetables rule

Vegetables whose leaves grow as a cross (cruciferous) are all part of a special food family that enhances the liver's capacity to detoxify. This includes cabbage, cauliflower, broccoli, Brussels sprouts and kale. They are good for us because they contain something called glucosinolates and D-glucarate that help a critical liver detox process called glucuronidation. To illustrate this, some ingenious scientists man-aged to extract the glucosinolates from Brussels sprouts and fed volunteers either regular Brussels sprouts that still contained gluco- sinolates, or those with it extracted. Those fed the glucosinolate-containing Brussels sprouts had a 30 per cent more active antioxidant-enzyme function, showing just how powerful these glucosinolates are.[7] That's why I recommend them, and, if you follow the recipes and menu plans, you'll be having a serving of cruciferous vegetables every day.

> ## CRUCIFEROUS VEGETABLES
>
> Have a serving of broccoli, Brussels sprouts, cabbage, cauliflower or kale every day.

## 4 Sulphur so good

Onions, spring onions, garlic and shallots are excellent food sources of sulphur-containing amino acids. Sulphur drives a critical liver detox pathway, called sulphation. The amino acids in these foods also give the body the raw ingredients to make glutathione, which drives another critical detox pathway. (You may recall that paracetamol and caffeine are detoxified by glutathione, page 23.) Red onions are especially good because they are high in quercetin, which is a natural anti-inflammatory, curbing allergic reactions and pain.

Garlic has many other benefits, a key one being as a gut protector. It's a natural antifungal agent, thereby helping to keep your digestive tract free of unwanted fungi and yeast.

### SULPHUR-UP YOUR DIET

Have a garlic clove, a small onion, shallot or four spring onions every day.

## 5 Get juicy

I want you to have a super-juice every day made from super-fruits. Super-fruits are high in antioxidants to support your liver, high in folic acid (which helps methylation, one of the most vital detoxification processes), high in zinc (vital for health and detoxification) and low in sugar. Blueberries, strawberries and raspberries are the best all-round foods for anti-ageing antioxidants compared to other fruit. A serving of strawberries contains more antioxidant power than three apples or four bananas. Best of all are blueberries, which are especially rich in a type of flavonoid called anthocyanidins and proanthocyanidins. You can measure the total antioxidant power of a food by its ability to detoxify oxygen radicals (oxidants). This is called the ORAC (Oxygen Radical Absorption Capacity) score. The higher the score the more potent the antioxidant. Berries come out on top, but there are other good fruits, too, including oranges, grapes and watermelon.

| Fruits | Zinc | Folic acid | ORAC | Vitamin C | Total ORAC score |
|---|---|---|---|---|---|
| Strawberries | 4 | 3 | 4 | 5 | 21 |
| Raspberries | 2 | 3 | 4 | 5 | 19 |
| Blueberries | 3 | 5 | 5 | 1 | 19 |
| Watermelon | 5 | 2 | 3 | 4 | 18 |
| Grapefruit | 0 | 4 | 3 | 5 | 16 |
| Oranges | 0 | 4 | 3 | 5 | 15 |
| Grapes | 4 | 5 | 2 | 2 | 14 |

**The top antioxidant fruits**

We've devised a selection of super-fruit smoothies based on these fruits for you. For example, there's the Berry Tasty, made with a handful of berries plus tahini, or my favourite, Watermelon Whizz, made simply by blending the flesh and seeds of a watermelon. The seeds crack and the black husk of the seed sinks to the bottom; the seed itself, which is rich in zinc, selenium, vitamin E and essential fats, becomes part of the drink with the vitamin C and beta-carotene-rich flesh. When berries are out of season you can use frozen berries, otherwise it's best to pick fresh, organic fruits.

## Add some carrot!

Although not a fruit, carrots are good combined with fruits for juices and smoothies. Carrots are great for you, and delicious with some apple or pear, and with ginger. Ginger is good for the digestion and a natural anti-inflammatory food. Try our Stomach Settler, made with carrot, pear, ginger, lemon juice and a little pineapple, which contains the digestive enzyme bromelain.

You can also make vegetable juices if you prefer, but ideally have a juice containing carrot, and a juice containing berries or watermelon every other day if you haven't eaten these foods already during the day (we have added a reminder on your menu plan for each day).

## Why make juices and smoothies?

The advantage of juicing or blending over actually eating the fruit or vegetable is that you can consume a greater variety – and variety is really the key to antioxidants. They work best when you take many different ones together. If you didn't juice, you would have to eat an awful lot of different fruits and vegetables to get the same level of plant nutrients. There are other advantages too: would you ever consider eating raw broccoli? Probably not, but it is a powerhouse of nutrients to support Phase 2 detoxification, and these are far more concentrated in its raw state than if it were cooked. A few stems of raw broccoli (Tenderstem is best) can be juiced easily or blended, and they combine easily with carrot and celery to make a delicious drink. Furthermore, if you use a blender, you can include parts of the fruit or vegetable that would otherwise be thrown away, such as the seeds and rind, where these amazing nutrients are most concentrated. If the end result is too thick to be a proper juice, then have it as a cold soup with a drizzle of bio-yoghurt and a sprig of mint. Think gazpacho.

> ## DRINK A SUPERFOOD JUICE OR SMOOTHIE EVERY DAY
>
> Choose from our menu of delicious smoothies, including berries, watermelon and citrus fruits (see page 148).

## Sugar in fruit

You might have noticed that the government guidelines on taking five portions of fruit and vegetables a day say that fruit juice counts as only one portion. This is because of the high sugar content of many fruits, particularly bananas, bearing in mind that the typical

British diet is already very high in sugar. However, your detox lasts only nine days and you will have removed your other sources of sugar during this time. Also, I believe the benefits of the vitamins and minerals contained in the fruit outweigh the temporary downside of the fruit sugar. But if you prefer not to add to your sugar load, avoid banana and stick to berries, or make it a vegetable juice.

# Maximise your intake of anti-ageing antioxidants ✅

I talked in Chapter 1 about the potential damage caused by oxidants (free radicals) and I also mentioned that we have means of neutralising them. This is where antioxidants come in. Some of these are made in the body and others are provided in our food. You've probably heard of the main food-derived antioxidants already: vitamin A (beta-carotene), vitamin C, vitamin E, zinc, selenium – and there are many others. Many of the steps you'll take on your 9-Day Liver Detox will greatly increase your intake of antioxidants, and the recipes and menus we have created take your antioxidant intake from food to the max.

Antioxidants are team players, as you can see in the illustration opposite, which shows how your body would disarm the oxidant from a French fry. It would need vitamin E (from seeds and fish), co-enzyme Q10 (mainly made in the body), vitamin C (from fruits and vegetables), glutathione (from onions and garlic) and anthocyanidins (from berries), with some beta-carotene (from carrots or watercress) and some alpha lipoic acid (made in the body) thrown in. Now you understand why these foods are all part of your 9-Day Liver Detox.

## How the antioxidants work

What's happening is something like 'pass the parcel' except that the parcel, the oxidant, is more like a hot potato. The antioxidant, vitamin E, for example, is like an oven glove and stops the oxidant from

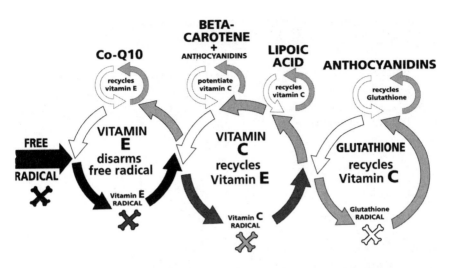

**Antioxidants are team players**

A fat-based oxidant, technically called a free radical, can be disarmed by vitamin E. The vitamin E molecule becomes an oxidant or free radical and is in turn disarmed and put back to work by vitamin C and CoQ10.

burning you. However, the antioxidant becomes hot in the process and itself becomes an oxidant. Ultimately, if you've got enough nutrients you'll quench the oxidant and reload the antioxidants to go back to work ready to disarm the next oxidant.

The box on the following page lists the top 20 antioxidant-rich foods, as rated on the ORAC scale (Oxygen Radical Absorption Capacity). Make sure you eat five of the 20 foods each day.

# Take detoxifying supplements ✅

In Chapter 1 we learned about a whole host of nutrients that make Phase 1 and Phase 2 of liver detoxification work best. Whereas the 9-Day Liver Detox will work in its own right, you can further improve and support your liver's ability to detoxify by supplementing the right combination of nutrients. On page 65, I recommend supplements for you to take only during your detox. You don't need to take them every day once the detox is over.

## THE TOP 20 ANTIOXIDANT POWER FOODS

All foods are in ORAC units per 100 grams (the higher the units the higher the antioxidants).

| | | |
|---|---|---|
| 1. | Pomegranate | 3,037 |
| 2. | Blueberries | 2,234 |
| 3. | Blackberries | 2,036 |
| 4. | Kale | 1,770 |
| 5. | Strawberries | 1,536 |
| 6. | Baby spinach, raw | 1,210 |
| 7. | Raspberries | 1,227 |
| 8. | Broccoli (Tenderstem) | 1,183 |
| 9. | Plums | 949 |
| 10. | Alfalfa sprouts | 931 |
| 11. | Spinach, steamed | 888 |
| 12. | Beetroot | 841 |
| 13. | Avocado | 782 |
| 14. | Orange | 750 |
| 15. | Grapes, red | 739 |
| 16. | Peppers, red | 731 |
| 17. | Cherries | 670 |
| 18. | Kiwi fruit | 602 |
| 19. | Beans, baked | 503 |
| 20. | Grapefruit, pink | 483 |

My first recommendation is to supplement a combination of digestive enzymes, probiotics and glutamine. Digestive enzymes digest your food, minimising the chances of whole food proteins getting into the blood. Probiotics are essential beneficial bacteria, which also play a part in the digestive process. I like the strains Lactobacillus acidophilus and Bifidobacteria. You don't need these every day of your life but a nine-day course is a great way to repopulate your gut flora or 'inner garden'. The combination of digestive enzymes plus probiotics, available in some supplements, is like a day at a health spa for your insides (see Resources).

My second recommendation is a further teaspoon of glutamine powder last thing at night to help maintain the integrity of the gut wall, your first line of defence from toxins (see Resources). Glutamine is direct fuel for the gut lining.

My third recommendation is an all-round antioxidant or liver-support formula (see Resources). Pick a formula that has as many of the key liver support nutrients shown below:

Vitamin C

Vitamin E

Coenzyme Q10

Glutathione

N-Acetyl Cysteine

Alpha Lipoic Acid

Glycine

Glutamine

Calcium-D-glucarate

Milk thistle (silymarin)

DIM (broccoli extract)

MSM (a form of sulphur)

Trimethyl Glycine (TMG)

In addition you need B vitamins that help methylation, but you'll find these, as well as basic levels of antioxidants plus minerals, in a high-potency multivitamin–mineral. I recommend everyone to take three basic supplements every day:

- A high potency multivitamin and mineral (good ones have 5mg zinc, 100mg magnesium)

- One gram of vitamin C, plus bioflavonoids found in berry extracts

- Essential omega-3 (EPA and DHA) and omega-6 (GLA) fats

Very rarely I have come across someone who is in such toxic overload that supplements and herbs can cause a bad reaction, such as headaches or nausea. If this is the case for you, then stop taking any supplements and just focus on the other food recommendations. You may have to do my 9-Day Liver Detox a couple of times before your body can tolerate the supplements.

## Take Detox Supplements Every Day

Your daily supplement programme should look like this:

| | Dosage | | |
| --- | --- | --- | --- |
| | **Breakfast** | **Lunch** | **Dinner** |
| **During the 9 Day-Liver Detox:** | | | |
| Digestive enzymes/probiotics | 1 | 1 | 1 |
| Glutamine powder | | | 1 tsp last thing |
| Antioxidant/liver support formula | 1 | 1 | |
| **Every day:** | | | |
| High potency multivitamin | 1 | 1 | |
| Vitamin C | 1 | 1 | |
| Essential fats (EPA, DHA and GLA) | 1 | | |

# Do detoxifying exercises every day ✅

Detoxification is about eliminating what is unnecessary. This is not only a process that happens in your body but is also a process for your mind and the environment you live in. In Chapter 1 I talked about unprocessed toxins being stored in the fat cells and eventually being released, detoxified and removed from the body via the blood, kidneys, gut and also the lymphatic system. The lymphatic system carries fats absorbed from food into the circulation and carries cellular waste (including stored toxins) to the liver for detoxification, so its efficient functioning is vital for your 9-Day Liver Detox. Unlike the cardiovascular system, which includes the heart, the lymphatic system doesn't have a pump and relies on movement to help detoxify. That's why breathing and physical exercise that stimulates lymphatic drainage help detoxification.

But exercise has another important role to play, and that is the generation of vital energy, called *chi* in Chinese medicine and *ki* in Japan. Any whole-body exercise is good for detoxification (brisk walking, jogging, swimming, yoga, and so on) but my favourite vital-energy-generating exercise is Psychocalisthenics because it combines both movement and *chi*-generating breathing.

Psychocalisthenics is a precise sequence of 23 exercises that leave you feeling fantastic. I've been using it for 20 years and I've yet to find anything that makes me feel better – which isn't bad for 15 minutes a day! Each exercise is driven by the breath, leaving you feeling lighter, freer and thoroughly oxygenated after a simple routine, which anyone can do. At first glance it looks like a powerful kind of aerobic yoga. Psychocalisthenics is designed to generate both physical fitness and vital energy by bringing mind and body into balance. It's key lies in the precise breathing pattern that accompanies each physical exercise.

The best way to learn Psychocalisthenics is to do a short course. For details see www.patrickholford.com/psychocalisthenics. You can also teach yourself from a DVD, but it is best to learn it in a class (see Resources).

Alternatively, join a yoga class that teaches breathing techniques (see Resources) and combine this with physical exercise such as walking for 20 minutes a day for a similar effect.

## Detoxifying breathing and meditation

Another way to generate vital energy is with meditation. This also helps to clear and detoxify the mind of endless thoughts. If you are new to meditation, I recommend a very simple breathing exercise, called Diakath breathing, which helps to deepen your breath, at the same time oxygenating the body while focusing the mind. Simply by doing this for five minutes a day you will be both meditating and generating vital energy.

This breathing exercise (reproduced opposite with the kind permission of Oscar Ichazo), connects the *kath* point – the body's centre of equilibrium – with the diaphragm muscle, so that deep breathing becomes natural and effortless. You can practise it at any time, while sitting, standing or lying down, and for as long as you like although, ideally, find somewhere quiet first thing in the morning. You can also do it unobtrusively during moments of stress. It is an excellent natural relaxant and energy booster, helping you to feel more connected and in tune.

The diaphragm is a dome-shaped muscle attached to the bottom of the rib cage. The *kath* is not an anatomical point like the navel, but is an energy point located in the lower belly, about three finger-widths below the navel. When you remember this point, you become aware of your entire body.

As you inhale, you will expand your lower belly from the *kath* point and your diaphragm muscle. This allows the lungs to fill with air from the bottom to the top. As you exhale, the belly and the diaphragm muscle relax, allowing the lungs to empty from top to bottom. Inhale and exhale through your nose.

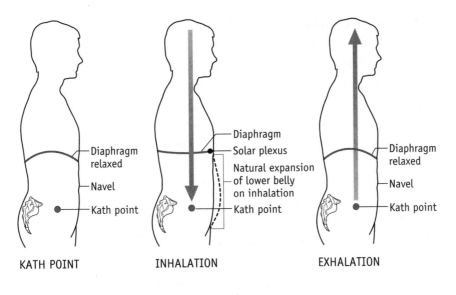

KATH POINT     INHALATION     EXHALATION

**Diakath breathing**

1 Sit comfortably, in a quiet place with your spine straight, in any one of the positions shown above.

2 Focus your attention in your *kath* point.

3 Let your belly expand from the *kath* point as you inhale slowly, deeply and effortlessly. Feel your diaphragm being pulled down towards the *kath* point as your lungs fill with air from the bottom to the top. On the exhale, relax both your belly and your diaphragm, emptying your lungs from top to bottom.

4 Repeat at your own pace.

5 Every morning, sit down in a quiet place before breakfast and practise Diakath breathing for a few minutes.

6 Whenever you are stressed throughout the day check your breathing. Practise Diakath breathing for nine breaths. This is great to do before an important meeting, or when something has upset you.

## Have a detoxifying massage

The body stores chemical toxins, physical tension and negative emotions. A good massage helps to detoxify at every level by stimulating the circulation and lymphatic system, and mobilising toxins. Regular massage is part of my ongoing strategy for detoxifying your life. Make sure you have one or two during your 9-Day Liver Detox.

## Detoxify your life

Detoxification is about eliminating what is unnecessary. As you do this on the inside, by detoxifying your body, you can also detoxify your mind. For example, make a commitment to resolve an issue you have with someone. Write a comprehensive letter expressing all your negative feelings about their behaviour or attitudes, going through every emotionally charged incident with them, really letting rip, holding nothing back, telling them that you won't accept their negative projections. However, don't send it! Now write a letter detailing everything you like about them, how much you've learned from them, going through every incident you can recall where you felt uplifted and supported by them. Don't send this letter either. This simple exercise should make you clearer on what is the real issue you have with the other person and you will feel more able to talk it through and resolve it with them, rather than continuing to hold on to it.

Also, why not detoxify the environment in which you live as well? Spring-clean a room in your house or workplace – perhaps your living room, bedroom, study or office. Go through each drawer and cupboard and throw away those items that you never use. If in doubt, throw it out. Now open the windows to air the room well and then clean your room thoroughly. Buy some flowers or a plant for your room and then burn some incense or aromatherapy oil.

# CHAPTER FOUR

# Test Your Detox Potential – Before and After

So that you can chart your own progress, it's a good idea to rate your detox potential before and after the 9-Day Liver Detox. There are two ways you can do this: with my simple Detox Check questionnaire, and with a more objective Detoxification Capacity Profile. The point of checking before and after is to demonstrate the difference that even a 9-Day Liver Detox can have on your life. If you score low on the Detox Check to start with, you at least have the satisfaction of knowing that your liver is now better able to cope with future toxins. Doing this detox even a couple of times a year will help prevent the many chronic degenerative diseases that plague modern life, such as heart disease, diabetes and arthritis.

## Using the Detoxification Capacity Profile

The Detoxification Capacity Profile involves a test kit that you order by post. It explains exactly what to do and involves you taking a urine sample. The advantage of the test is that it does help you fine-tune your supplement programme. This is particularly helpful for people with chronic digestive problems or fatigue.

The test involves you swallowing a measured amount of caffeine, paracetamol and aspirin in a pill. You then collect your urine sample (the kit provides a container) and you'll get a report that looks like this:

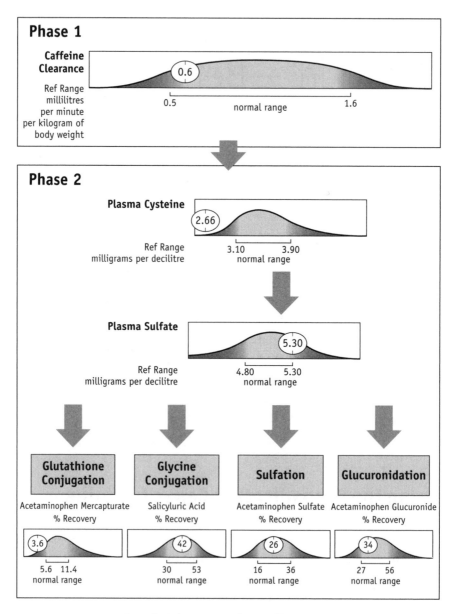

**A typical detox capacity profile report**

## Looking at the profile report

As I described in Chapter 1, Phase 1 is where toxins are worked on by P450 enzymes to prepare them for Phase 2. This person's Phase 1 is just within normal range but is verging on sluggish, so they would benefit from the vitamins and minerals that would help boost Phase-1 detoxification (see Chapter 1 page 22).

Phase 2 is where toxins from Phase 1 are 'conjugated' to make them non-toxic. This person has extremely low plasma cysteine, which is used to make glutathione for glutathione conjugation. Consequently, you can see that glutathione conjugation is similarly below normal range. They would benefit from eating more onions and garlic, nuts and seeds for selenium (to help manufacture the glutathione enzymes) and supplementing N-acetyl-cysteine or glutathione (and eating berries to improve their utilisation). This person's plasma sulphate is high, and consequently sulphation is working normally. Glycine conjugation and glucuronidation are similarly normal.

If you'd like to be guided by a test like this see Resources on page 172 to order a test kit. It also gives you the option to retest yourself to see how you've improved your liver detox function.

## The Detox Check questionnaires

Below are four questionnaires that make up my Detox Check. One covers **energy**, the next **digestion**, then **detox** and finally **aches and pains**. Each question gives you three possible scores (0, 1 or 2).

**Score 0** if you never or rarely have this symptom; for example, less than once a month

**Score 1** if you sometimes have this symptom; for example, more than once a month

**Score 2** if you either always or frequently have this symptom; for example, at least every week

So, your worst possible score is 80. Score yourself in the 'Now' column, as an average for the last week. Once you've finished your 9-Day Liver Detox, score yourself again.

## QUESTIONNAIRE energy check

| | Now | After detox |
|---|---|---|
| 1. Are you rarely wide awake within 15 minutes of rising? | 2 | |
| 2. Do you need tea, coffee, a cigarette or something sweet to get you going in the morning? | 2 | |
| 3. Do you crave chocolate, sweet foods, bread, cereal or pasta? | 1 | |
| 4. Do you add sugar to your drinks, have sugared drinks or add sugared sauces, such as ketchup, to your food? | 1 | |
| 5. Do you often have energy slumps during the day or after meals? | 1 | |
| 6. Do you crave something sweet or a stimulant after meals? | 0 | |
| 7. Do you often have mood swings or difficulty concentrating? | 2 | |
| 8. Do you get dizzy or irritable if you go six hours without food? | 2 | |
| 9. Do you find you over-react to stress? | 2 | |
| 10. Is your energy now less than it used to be? | 2 | |
| 11. Do you feel too tired to exercise? | 2 | |
| **Your total energy score** | 17 | |

## QUESTIONNAIRE digestion check

|  | Now | After detox |
|---|---|---|
| **1.** Do you get a burning sensation or feeling of indigestion in your stomach? | 1 | |
| **2.** Do you use indigestion tablets? | 2 | |
| **3.** Do you often have an uncomfortable feeling of fullness in your stomach? | 2 | |
| **4.** Do you find it difficult digesting fatty foods? | 0 | |
| **5.** Do you often get diarrhoea? | 1 | |
| **6.** Do you often suffer from constipation? | 1 | |
| **7.** Do you often get a bloated stomach? | 0 | |
| **8.** Do you often feel nauseous? | 0 | |
| **9.** Do you often belch or pass wind? | 1 | |
| **10.** Do you fail to have a bowel movement at least once a day? | 0 | |
| **Your total digestion score** | 8 | |

## QUESTIONNAIRE detox check

|  | Now | After detox |
|---|---|---|
| **1.** Do you suffer from bad breath? | 0 | |
| **2.** Do you have watery or itchy eyes or swollen, red or sticky eyelids, bags or dark circles under your eyes? | 1 | |
| **3.** Do you have itchy ears, earache, ear infections, drainage from the ear or ringing in the ears? | 0 | |

4. Do you suffer from excessive mucus, a stuffy nose or sinus problems?  `2`

5. Do you suffer from acne, skin rashes or hives?  `2`

6. Do you sweat a lot and have a strong body odour, including your feet?  `2`

7. Do you have a sluggish metabolism and find it hard to lose weight, or are you underweight and find it hard to gain weight?  `2`

8. Do you have a bitter taste in your mouth or a furry tongue?  `0`

9. Do you easily get a hangover and feel considerably worse the next day even after a small amount of alcohol?  `2`

10. Does coffee leave you feeling jittery or unwell?  `1`

**Your total detox score**  `12`

## QUESTIONNAIRE pain check

|  | Now | After detox |
|---|---|---|

1. Do you suffer from headaches or migraine?  `2`

2. Do you suffer from allergies?  `2`

3. Do you have joint or muscle aches or pains?  `2`

4. Do you suffer from IBS (irritable bowel syndrome)?  `0`

5. Do you suffer from hayfever?  `1`

6. Do you suffer from rashes, itches, eczema or dermatitis?  `0`

7. Do you suffer from asthma or shortness of breath? ☐ ☐

8. Do you suffer from colitis, diverticulitis or Crohn's disease? ☐ ☐

9. Do you suffer from other aches or pains? ☐ ☐

10. Do you use painkillers most weeks? ☐ ☐

**Your total pain score** ☐ ☐

## Score

Now add up your total scores and fill them in below:

**Energy** ___ + **Digestion** ___ + **Detox** ___ + **Pain** ___ = ___

Ideally, what you want is a score of no more than 2 in any section and not more than 10 in total. Whatever your score is now, what's important is your score after your 9-Day Liver Detox.

Your total 'after' score: _____

### Above 30 (and has decreased by one-third during detox)

If your score is above 30 and has decreased by a third or more during your 9-Day Liver Detox, keep going. You need to continue with these detox principles for a month.

### Above 30 (without much change during detox)

If your score is above 30 and hasn't changed much during your 9-Day Liver Detox, have you been taking the recommended supplements? As well as continuing with the detox principles, see a nutritional therapist, who can advise you in more detail and, if necessary, run some tests to find out why you feel under par.

### Between 10 and 29

If your score has decreased substantially and is between 10 and 29, well done. You are making progress and now need to integrate as many of these principles as you can into your daily life. Rescore yourself again after 90 days.

**Below 10**

You are in reasonably good health. Well done. You may choose to do an annual 9-Day Liver Detox – especially if this made a big difference to how you feel – or you may wish to incorporate as many of these principles into your daily life.

---

### HAVE YOU COMPLETED YOUR 9-DAY DETOX DIET?

How did you do? Can you spare three minutes to let us know? Go online at www.patrickholford.com/detoxtest and help with our research. Let us know:

- Your before and after score

- Reasons for doing the 9-Day Liver Detox Diet

- How your health has changed and

- What you have learnt.

You'll be helping us to research, refine and improve the detox process at the same time.

---

In Chapter 7 I explain how to maintain your health improvements and detox for life.

# PART TWO

# CHAPTER **FIVE**

# Start Detoxing Now!

Your 9-Day Liver Detox is designed to be followed over two weekends, with one whole week in between. You really need the full nine days for the detox improvement to start showing up in feelings of well-being and the lessening of symptoms. The idea of the two weekends sandwiched around a full week is that it will make life as easy for you as possible in terms of shopping, preparing and implementing the diet if you are working full time. This gives you some time to get used to the new way of eating without the pressures and time constraints of work. If this isn't convenient, however, feel free to start whenever it suits you.

Fiona and I are going to tell you exactly what to do, down to providing your exact shopping list. The first thing you need to do is set the date – as soon as possible. Remember: tomorrow is the most special day. Why? Because everything always happens tomorrow! So, get your diary out now and make a date. It's important to pick a week and weekends where you won't be under pressure to drink or eat vast amounts of food. It's even better if you can pick a week when you are in an environment that supports your transformation to a new you.

You will need the following for your detox, and these are itemised later in this chapter:

**Food** You will find complete shopping lists to see you through the detox period (see pages 92–101).

**Supplements** See Chapter 3 for a full explanation of the supplements I suggest you take and page 104 for a chart listing when to take them.

**Good-quality water** In Chapter 3 I explained how important it is to drink plenty of water, either bottled or filtered. On page 53 we list the requirements for your detox, as a reminder while you gather everything together in preparation.

You will also need to be clear about the rules, because following them will give you the best transformation. On pages 84–6 is a complete list of what you'll be eating and avoiding, which incorporates all the points from Chapters 2 and 3.

We have given you an exact 9-Day Menu Plan, with details of all the recipes. Alternatively, you could create your own plan based on foods from the 'included' list on pages 85–6. However, if you choose your own foods from the 'included' list, you also need to ensure that you follow my Six Golden Liver-detox Rules listed in the box opposite.

Following our 9-Day Menu Plan is easier than doing it yourself, because we have integrated all of the golden rules into the daily menus. Have a look now on pages 87–92 so that you have a sense of what a typical day looks like.

You'll notice that most of the instructions are obvious, but some link through to precise recipes when there's something you have to make. The 9-Day Menu Plan is followed by your Shopping List. You need to go shopping twice during your detox – on Day 1 (Saturday), or the day before, and on Day 4 (Thursday).

That's it. The following pages give you everything you need to know:

Pages 84–6      What to avoid and what to eat

Pages 87–92     Your 9-Day Menu Plan

Pages 92–101    Your Shopping Lists

Pages 102–3     Preparing for the Six Golden Liver-detox Rules

Pages 103–4     Your liver-detox Supplement Support Programme

## THE SIX GOLDEN LIVER-DETOX RULES

1. Drink eight glasses of water or fluid every day (see Chapter 3 and page 85).

2. Have a tablespoon of ground seeds every day (see Chapter 3 and page 85).

3. Have a serving of our Super Greens Mix every day (see Chapter 3 and page 86).

4. Have a serving of cruciferous vegetables (broccoli, Brussels sprouts, cabbage, cauliflower or kale) every day (see Chapter 3 and page 86).

5. Have a garlic clove, a small onion, shallot or four spring onions every day for their sulphur content (see Chapter 3 and page 86).

6. Have one of our superfood juices or smoothies every day (see Chapter 3 and page 86).

# What to avoid and what to eat

In Chapters 2 and 3 we listed the Five Habits to Break and the Five Habits to Make. Here is a reminder of those foods for you to see at a glance.

## Foods to avoid

Avoid all the following foods and drinks, as explained in Chapter 2:

**Wheat** You will have to avoid bread made from wheat and all commercially made cakes, biscuits, pastries and pasta. Also, check the labels of all other commercially made foods to ensure that no wheat is included. Instead, buy non-wheat (and preferably gluten-free) alternatives or make your own from non-gluten flour (available in health-food stores and good supermarkets). (See pages 31–6 for a full explanation of the problems with wheat on a detox.)

**Milk** You will have to avoid milk from any animal source, cheese, cream, butter, ice cream, yoghurt, probiotic drinks such as Actimel or Yakult, and food with milk solids, whey or casein on the label. Instead, buy rice, almond, coconut or quinoa milk, coconut or pumpkin-seed butter, or tahini or soya cream (or make your own with finely ground cashews and water), or any nut or seed butter (except peanut butter). (See pages 36–9 for a full explanation of the problems with milk on a detox.)

**Caffeine** You will have to avoid coffee, black tea, colas and diet colas, Red Bull and other caffeinated drinks. Remember to reduce coffee to a maximum of one cup a day before starting the detox, or you could be in for a ferocious headache. If you can give up al-together before starting, that would be even better. Please do not substitute the decaffeinated versions of these drinks, as they contain potential carcinogens that also have to be detoxified. Substitute up to two weak cups of green tea, rooibosch, herbal tea or water. (See pages 39–45 for a full explanation of the problems with caffeine on a detox.)

**Alcohol** Replace with mineral water or organic fruit juice. You can also try fruit smoothies as an alternative. (See pages 45–8 for a full explanation of the problems with alcohol on a detox.)

**Bad fats** You will have to avoid all meat, all fried food (including any vegetables, French fries and crisps), all processed foods containing hydrogenated (or partially hydrogenated) oils, commercial mayonnaise and all margarines and spreads. Substitute with essential fats from fish (but not fried fish), eggs, olive oil, raw nuts and seeds, and nut and seed butters and oils. (But don't cook with them; if you are intending to use oil in cooking, use only olive oil.) (See pages 48–50 for a full explanation of the problems with bad fats on a detox.)

## Essential foods

If you are not following the 9-Day Menu Plan on page 87, it is important that you stick rigidly to the Five Habits to Break and the Five Habits to Make. In accordance with these, we have put together a list of absolutely essential detox foods for you to stock up on:

**A large quantity of bottled water,** if you do not have a water filter. Bear in mind that you could be getting through 2 litres (3½ pints) a day. The detox potential is enhanced if you have a mug of hot water with the juice of half a lemon twice a day, as this encourages bile flow, which helps remove toxins. So, you will also need nine lemons.

**Pumpkin, sunflower and sesame seeds, and flax seeds,** which contain the omega-3 and omega-6 essential fats to help repair damaged cell membranes. They are also rich in the minerals needed for the detoxification and antioxidant enzymes. You will need enough for one tablespoon a day.

**Dark green leafy vegetables** (baby spinach, watercress, basil, parsley). These vegetables are rich in vitamin C, folate, chlorophyll and antioxidants. They are best eaten raw in a salad, as cooking destroys their vitamin content.

**Cruciferous vegetables** (brassicas), comprising broccoli (Tenderstem is particularly good), Brussels sprouts, cabbage, cauliflower, kale, turnip, kohlrabi. These contain a number of essential compounds that help support detoxification. So that you will not lose the benefits of all the vitamins, steam or lightly stir-fry only or try adding raw broccoli (Tenderstem, if possible) to vegetable juices.

**Onions** (especially red), spring onions, shallots and garlic. These produce the sulphur necessary for the detoxification process and can reduce inflammation. Again, eat raw if you can!

**Make a vegetable juice** with any of the vegetables mentioned above and experiment with adding carrots, mixed peppers, tomatoes, celery and apples, which are all high in antioxidants. The pectin in apples helps transport toxins out of the body.

**Make a fruit juice** with any combination of berries (especially strawberries, blueberries, raspberries) and pomegranates for their antioxidant properties.

**Get your protein from eggs and oily fish** (salmon, trout, herring, pilchards, mackerel, sardines, anchovies and fresh tuna – but eat tuna only once during the nine days, as it contains heavy metals). Eggs are the purest form of protein, and they also contain sulphur for detoxification, whereas oily fish is rich in omega-3 essential fats. Have the eggs boiled to avoid adding any fats during cooking.

# Your 9-Day Menu Plan

The following menu plan is specifically designed with your new goals in mind – to make it easy to stick to your new habits to make (see Chapter 3) and to help you break the old habits (see Chapter 2). The dishes are jam-packed with superfoods, antioxidants and water to meet your daily goals, as well as being free from caffeine, alcohol, bad fats, wheat and milk. You can follow our menu plan here or come up with your own, following our guidelines (outlined on page 83). We have included some repeated recipes to allow you to batch-cook and save time.

## Day 1 (Saturday)

**Breakfast:** Superfood Muesli with Essential Seed Mix

**Morning snack:** 2 plums plus half a dozen almonds

**Lunch:** Superboost Sesame Salad

**Afternoon snack:** olives and your daily smoothie or juice

**Supper:** Fennel and Mixed Rice Pilaff with a large mixed salad

**Drinks:** one fresh juice or smoothie (ideally have a juice containing carrot, and a juice containing berries or watermelon every other day if you haven't eaten these foods already during the day), plus un-limited water, herbal teas and coffee alternatives

## Day 2 (Sunday)

**Breakfast:** Super-fruit and Seed Salad including Essential Seed Mix

**Morning snack:** Hummus with Crudités

**Lunch:** Trout en Papillote with Roasted Vegetables followed by Fruit Burst Frozen Yoghurt

**Afternoon snack:** pomegranate or grapefruit

**Supper:** Patrick's Primordial Soup – stir in a serving of Super Greens Mix

**Drinks:** one fresh juice or smoothie (ideally have a juice containing carrot, and a juice containing berries or watermelon every other day if you haven't eaten these foods already during the day), plus un- limited water, herbal teas and coffee alternatives

## At the end of Day 2

You may now be experiencing a few withdrawal symptoms from all the toxins you were consuming earlier: headache, nausea and possi- ble lightheadedness. These are nothing to worry about. Just remem- ber, there is a direct correlation between the withdrawal symptoms and the amount of toxins previously consumed.

# Day 3 (Monday)

**Breakfast:** Cinnamon Fruit Porridge including Essential Seed Mix

**Morning snack:** avocado with lemon juice

**Lunch:** Skin-defence Dip with rocket on pumpernickel-style rye bread

**Afternoon snack:** Corn on the Cob, plus your daily smoothie or juice

**Supper:** Age-defying Carrot and Lentil Soup (make double quantities for supper tomorrow). Stir in a serving of Super Greens Mix

**Drinks:** one fresh juice or smoothie (ideally have a juice containing carrot, and a juice containing berries or watermelon every other day if you haven't eaten these foods already during the day), plus un- limited water, herbal teas and coffee alternatives

# Day 4 (Tuesday)

**Breakfast:** Berry Breakfast Smoothie

**Morning snack:** Hummus with Crudités

**Lunch:** Age-defying Carrot and Lentil Soup (left over from yesterday)

**Afternoon snack:** apple plus a handful of walnuts

**Supper:** Rice with Super-greens Pesto

**Drinks:** one fresh juice or smoothie (ideally have a juice containing carrot, and a juice containing berries or watermelon every other day if you haven't eaten these foods already during the day), plus unlimited water, herbal teas and coffee alternatives

## At the end of Day 4

By now I would expect all the withdrawal symptoms to have passed, and you will now be settling into the new routine of healthy eating. Remember, you never have to go hungry. Eat as much as you like of all the permitted foods.

# Day 5 (Wednesday)

**Breakfast:** Super-fruit and Seed Salad including Essential Seed Mix

**Morning snack:** pear with a handful of pecan nuts

**Lunch:** Superfood Sandwich for Beautiful Skin, including Super Greens Mix

**Afternoon snack:** Guacamole with Crudités

**Supper:** Leek, Cannellini and Potato Soup (double up on the quantities for supper tomorrow)

**Drinks:** one fresh juice or smoothie (ideally have a juice containing carrot, and a juice containing berries or watermelon every other day if you haven't eaten these foods already during the day), plus unlimited water, herbal teas and coffee alternatives

# Day 6 (Thursday)

**Breakfast:** Superfood Muesli including Essential Seed Mix

**Morning snack:** toasted pumpkin and sunflower seeds, plus a piece of fruit, if you like

**Lunch:** Leek, Cannellini and Potato Soup (left over from yesterday) – stir in a serving of Super Greens Mix

**Afternoon snack:** Hummus with Crudités

**Supper:** Cleansing Bean and Artichoke Salad

**Drinks:** one fresh juice or smoothie (ideally have a juice containing carrot, and a juice containing berries or watermelon every other day if you haven't eaten these foods already during the day), plus unlimited water, herbal teas and coffee alternatives

## At the end of Day 6

Well done for sticking to the healthy-eating regime this far. You have now been on the detox diet for almost a week and I would expect some of the benefits to become apparent: increased energy, more refreshed on waking, fewer energy dips during the day.

# Day 7 (Friday)

**Breakfast:** Cinnamon Fruit Porridge with a serving of Essential Seed Mix

**Morning snack:** nectarine (or other seasonal fruit) with a handful of cashew nuts

**Lunch:** Superboost Sesame Salad

**Afternoon snack:** olives, plus a piece of fruit, if you like

**Supper:** Baked Sweet Potatoes with Borlotti Stew

**Drinks:** one fresh juice or smoothie (ideally have a juice containing carrot, and a juice containing berries or watermelon every other day if you haven't eaten these foods already during the day), plus unlimited water, herbal teas and coffee alternatives

# Day 8 (Saturday)

**Breakfast:** Toast and Nut Butter

**Morning snack:** apple, plus a handful of cashew nuts

**Lunch:** Raw Summer Soup (or one of the hot soups, if out of season) – stir in a serving of Super Greens Mix

**Afternoon snack:** raw baby corn with Hummus

**Supper:** Mushroom and Pine Nut Stuffed Peppers with a large mixed salad

**Drinks:** one fresh juice or smoothie (ideally have a juice containing carrot, and a juice containing berries or watermelon every other day if you haven't eaten these foods already during the day), plus unlimited water, herbal teas and coffee alternatives

# Day 9 (Sunday)

**Breakfast:** Berry Breakfast Smoothie including Essential Seed Mix

**Morning snack:** Roasted Pumpkin Seeds

**Lunch:** Salmon with Puy Lentils followed by Detox Pear and Blueberry Crumble

**Afternoon snack:** olives, plus your daily smoothie or juice

**Supper:** Superfood Salad of Quinoa with Roasted Vegetables, including Super Greens Mix

**Drinks:** one fresh juice or smoothie (ideally have a juice containing carrot, and a juice containing berries or watermelon every other day if you haven't eaten these foods already during the day), plus unlimited water, herbal teas and coffee alternatives

## At the end of Day 9

Congratulations! You have now completed my 9-Day Liver Detox. I hope you are now seeing and feeling the benefits of all the health and energy improvements. But even if they are not all that you had hoped for, you can at least know that you have done a significant amount to ward off the many degenerative diseases that can result from an overloaded liver.

But please do not relapse into all your old habits now, however comfortable. How about making one of my detox diet changes permanent, such as eating broccoli several times a week or reducing drinking coffee by one cup per day and substituting a herbal tea. Then, when you come to repeat my 9-Day Liver Detox, it will be all the easier for you.

# Your Shopping Lists

It is worth stocking up on the following foods to help you follow the nine-day plan. This will also save extra trips to the supermarket during the week when temptation might lead you to the chocolate aisle! You can find all the items in good supermarkets and health-food stores.

## Shopping list on Day 1
(for example, Saturday) or the day before

Read through the recipes in Chapter 6 before making your list in case you want to make any adjustments to suit your personal preferences, but remember to keep to healthy alternatives as explained in Chapter 3 and in this chapter.

**Vegetables**

2 garlic bulbs

bag of red onions

bag of white onions

bag of baby spinach

pack of watercress

mixed salad leaves

pack of basil

head of celery

1 fennel bulb

large bag of carrots

box of mushrooms

small box chestnut mushrooms

1 aubergine

1 corn on the cob

2 avocados

2 medium or 1 large sweet potato

bunch of spring onions

2 courgettes

2 large sweet potatoes, or 4 small–medium ones

2 beetroot

small piece of fresh root ginger

a selection of two or three cruciferous vegetables, such as broccoli
   (Tenderstem, if possible), Brussels sprouts, cabbage, cauliflower
     or kale

pack of alfalfa sprouts

fresh flat-leaf parsley

fresh basil

## Fruit

2 pomegranates

bag of lemons

1 pink grapefruit

a few bananas (not too ripe)

1 watermelon

mango (optional)

kiwi fruit (optional)

1 large punnet of blueberries, or a small punnet of blueberries and
a small punnet of other berries such as raspberries

cherries

3 red peppers

2 plums

bag of apples

plus fruit and vegetables for juices and smoothies (see pages 151–3)

## Refrigerator

flax seeds (linseeds)

1 medium bag of pumpkin seeds, about 200g (7oz)

1 medium bag of sesame seeds, about 200g (7oz)

1 medium bag of sunflower seeds, about 200g (7oz)

1 medium bag of flaked almonds, about 200g (7oz)

2 medium-sized rainbow trout (if serving two people, otherwise
buy 1), preferably organic, fully prepared

large pot of soya yoghurt (choose an organic brand with no
added sugar)

2 large pots of hummus

## Freezer

1 bag, about 400g (14oz), frozen mixed berries (from the
supermarket)

## Store cupboard

large bag of whole rolled porridge oats

small bag of whole oat flakes

bag of brown rice (preferably basmati)

small bag of mixed rice (wild rice, brown basmati rice and red
Camargue rice)

packet of quinoa

small bag of pot or pearl barley

1 box rough oatcakes

bags of nuts (such as walnuts, pine nuts, almonds, hazelnuts, pecan
nuts, cashew nuts)

bag of ground almonds

bag of desiccated coconut

sun-blush tomatoes (optional)

1 jar of nut butter

1 jar of green olives

1 jar Kalamata olives

2 jars of marinated artichoke hearts

1 can chickpeas

2 cans borlotti beans

1 can green lentils

1 can tomatoes

1 can mixed pulses

2 cans chickpeas

bag of Puy lentils (dried)

bag of red split lentils (dried)

natural mineral water (if you don't have a water filter)

ground cinnamon

ground turmeric

black peppercorns

1 tub Marigold Reduced Salt Vegetable Bouillon powder

small tub of coconut oil or medium (not extra virgin) olive oil

small bottle cold pressed oil (extra virgin olive oil, or flax or
   hemp oil)

small bottle toasted sesame oil

(**Note** If you are worried about the initial outlay, stick to olive oil rather than the more expensive flax or hemp oils, and bear in mind that all of these ingredients can be easily used up after the detox has finished.)

can of coconut milk

carton of rice milk (optional)

tube of tomato purée

bag of xylitol (safe sugar alternative sourced from plants, available
   in good supermarkets and health-food stores)

plus caffeine-free alternatives (see below)

pumpernickel-style rye bread

**For smoothies** You will also need your chosen fruits and vegetables for juices and smoothies (see pages 151–3).

**Seeds and green leafy vegetables and herbs** You will need enough for your daily servings of Essential Seed Mix and the Super Greens Mix respectively (see the list on pages 93–6 and pages 109 and 122–3). You may need to stock up on these through the week, especially your fresh greens once you have decided which combinations you prefer.

## Drinks

Don't forget to try some of the following caffeine-free alternatives to tea and coffee:

**Herbal and fruit teas** such as peppermint and chamomile, lemon and ginger.

**Rooibosch (red bush) tea** This South African leaf tea is naturally caffeine-free and very popular with black-tea fans, as although it does not taste the same it has a similarly strong flavour and can be drunk with or without milk. On the 9-Day Liver Detox, substitute milk with soya or rice milk.

**Dandelion coffee** is a liver-friendly substitute for coffee, but don't expect it to taste like the real thing!

# Shopping List on Day 5
(for example, Wednesday)

Make sure you don't need to restock items such as nuts and seeds that you are eating every day.

## Vegetables

head of celery

bag of baby spinach

pack of watercress

mixed salad leaves

pack of alfalfa sprouts

more fresh basil and parsley if your supplies need topping up

fresh coriander

small bag or a handful of baby new potatoes

a selection of two or three cruciferous vegetables, such as broccoli
(Tenderstem, if possible), Brussels sprouts, cabbage, cauliflower
or kale

1 large sweet potato, or 2 small–medium ones, plus another
small one

1 corn on the cob

a few baby corn cobs

4 large red peppers

4 shallots (optional)

box mushrooms, about 140g (5oz)

bunch of spring onions

1 avocado

half a cucumber

6 large leeks

1 small courgette

900g (2lb) cherry tomatoes

### Fruit

small bunch of bananas (not too ripe)

about 3 large punnets of blueberries (buy a couple now and then
buy more as and when you need them, to avoid wastage)

1 pomegranate

3 pears

nectarine (or other seasonal fruit)

bag of apples

### Refrigerator

3 salmon fillets, preferably organic (if serving two people,
otherwise buy 2)

large pot of hummus

pot of guacamole (or an extra avocado to make your own)

You will also need to top up your supplies of fruit and vegetables for
juices and smoothies to see you through the remainder of the plan,
as well as oatcakes, lemons, carrots, onions and garlic, if you have
used up your supplies from earlier in the week.

# General Shopping List

If you are not following the 9-Day Menu Plan on page 87, we have put together a more general list of foods that are used in the recipes, for you to stock up on:

## Fresh foods

Assortment of fruit and vegetables according to your likes and what is in season or available. Here are some suggestions:

**Vegetables**

a selection of two or three cruciferous vegetables, such as broccoli (Tenderstem, if possible), Brussels sprouts, cabbage, cauliflower or kale

aubergine

avocados

baby spinach

basil

carrots

celery

fresh coriander

corn on the cob

baby corn

courgettes

flat-leaf parsley

fresh root ginger root

garlic

leeks

lettuce or mixed salad leaves

mixed peppers

mushrooms

red onions

sweet potatoes

tomatoes

watercress

white onions

## Fruit

apples

bananas

berries (for example, blueberries, strawberries and raspberries)

grapes

pink grapefruit

kiwi fruit

lemons

mango

oranges

pears

pomegranate

watermelon

## Refrigerator

hummus

guacamole (if not making your own)

soya yoghurt (choose an organic brand with no added sugar)

pumpkin or squash

sunflower, pumpkin and sesame seeds

200g (7oz) flax seeds (linseeds)

olives

salmon fillets

trout fillets

omega-rich seed-oil blend

**Freezer**

> peas
>
> frozen mixed berries

**Store cupboard**

> unsalted nut butter
>
> whole rolled porridge oats
>
> ground almonds
>
> tahini
>
> xylitol (safe sugar alternative sourced from plants, available in good supermarkets and health-food stores)
>
> coconut oil or second press (medium or mild) olive oil for cooking
>
> extra virgin olive oil
>
> toasted sesame oil
>
> canned mixed pulses
>
> canned or dried chickpeas
>
> canned or dried borlotti beans
>
> dried Puy lentils
>
> quinoa
>
> ground ginger
>
> ground cinnamon
>
> marinated artichoke hearts (in jars or from the deli)
>
> canned coconut milk
>
> rice milk
>
> pine nuts
>
> mixed nuts
>
> Marigold Reduced Salt Vegetable Bouillon powder
>
> tomato purée
>
> turmeric
>
> dried herbes de Provence or mixed dried herbs
>
> natural mineral water (if you don't have a water filter)

# Preparing for the Six Golden Liver-detox Rules

## 1 Drink eight glasses of water or fluid every day

This is the equivalent to 1.5 litres (2¾ pints) water, and can be drunk cold or hot, as in non-caffeine teas. Add half a lemon squeezed into a mug of hot water twice a day.

Choose either filtered water (see Resources page 170) or bottled natural mineral water.

## 2 Have a tablespoon of ground seeds every day

Seeds are incredibly rich in essential fats, minerals, vitamin E, protein and fibre. Make up our Essential Seed Mix (see page 109) to add to your cereal each day.

## 3 Have a serving of our Super Greens Mix every day

Each day make a Super Greens blend (see page 122) using a handful each of baby spinach leaves, watercress, parsley and basil, with variations, such as sun-blush tomatoes, artichoke hearts, pine nuts, pumpkin seeds and avocado.

## 4 Have a serving of cruciferous vegetables

Eat a serving of broccoli (Tenderstem is best), Brussels sprouts, cabbage, cauliflower or kale every day. These are ideally eaten raw or can be lightly steamed or stir-fried in a small amount of oil or try steam-frying.

> **STEAM-FRYING**
>
> Add about 2 tbsp of liquid (such as water, vegetable stock or a watered-down sauce) to a wok or large frying pan – use one with a lid. When the liquid is boiling, add your vegetables, stir-fry for about 1 minute then place the lid on the pan to allow the ingredients to steam inside. Turn down the heat after a couple of minutes and steam until the vegetables are al dente – you can always add a splash more water if the pan dries out.

## 5 Have a garlic clove, a small onion, shallot or four spring onions every day

Sulphur-up your diet with these health-giving vegetables each day. Eat them raw if possible.

## 6 Have one of our superfood juices or smoothies every day

Choose from our menu of delicious superfood juices and smoothies, which include refreshing and healthy fruits such as berries, watermelon and citrus fruits (see pages 151–3).

# Your liver-detox Supplement Support Programme

The following chart gives you the supplements to take during your 9-Day Liver Detox to get the best results. Remember to take detox supplements every day.

| | Dosage | | |
|---|---|---|---|
| | **Breakfast** | **Lunch** | **Dinner** |
| **During the 9 Day-Liver Detox:** | | | |
| Digestive enzymes/probiotics/glutamine | 1 | 1 | 1 |
| Glutamine powder | | | 1 tsp last thing |
| Antioxidant/liver support formula | 1 | 1 | |
| **Every day:** | | | |
| High potency multivitamin | 1 | 1 | |
| Vitamin C | 1 | 1 | |
| Essential fats (DHA, GLA and EPA) | 1 | | |

# Troubleshooting

Most people will have no trouble at all on this diet and will feel great by the end. Just occasionally, though, you might feel a bit rough at the beginning. Here is what might happen and what to do about it.

## Withdrawal symptoms

I have already talked about the need to reduce coffee to a maximum of one cup a day before starting the detox to minimise the risk of headaches. This is because caffeine is an addictive substance and you will be going through withdrawal. The same may also be true of any food you have given up (such as wheat and dairy) to which you are allergic or sensitive. You may not just have a headache, you may feel weak and nauseous as well, and you may find yourself craving the food (or caffeine) you have given up.

This is a very clear indication that you are indeed sensitive to these foods, and we would recommend that you cut them out of your diet completely for three months and then reintroduce them one at a time and very slowly. Unfortunately, there is nothing to be done about these symptoms except to drink even more water and to rest. They should pass in 24–36 hours.

Cravings can be combated to some extent by having a substitute food. For example, if you are craving dairy foods, nibble on mixed seeds or dip some bread into flax seed oil; this will provide you with an alternative fat but one that will only do you good. Sugar cravings can be reduced by taking a chromium supplement, giving 200mcg of chromium, or having a teaspoon of glutamine powder.

## Coated tongue, bad breath and body odour

Believe it or not, a coated tongue, bad breath or body odour are good signs, demonstrating that your body really is detoxing. They will pass after a few days.

Meanwhile, shower regularly but do not use soap, shower gel or deodorant unless they come from a health-food store and are free of toxic chemicals and heavy metals (deodorants usually contain aluminium). Clean your teeth regularly but gently (don't allow your gums to bleed), preferably with toothpaste that, similarly, does not contain fluoride or other toxic chemicals. Do not use mouthwash. Keep drinking water to encourage the toxins to leave your body in urine rather than sweat and saliva.

## Constipation or diarrhoea

You are unlikely to suffer from constipation because you will be eating so much more fibre and drinking so many more fluids. If it occurs it will just be the body's way of adjusting to your new eating habits. Don't take any laxatives. It will pass quickly.

Diarrhoea is more common and is just the result of the additional fibre combined with the body adjusting to not having the usual constipating proteins and refined carbohydrates. However, you lose additional fluids when you have diarrhoea, so be sure to drink even more water. The diarrhoea should pass in a couple of days but if it does not, then leave out all nuts and seeds and cut out vitamin C supplements until you pass normally formed stools, then resume.

Be aware that the number of bowel movements in a day will almost certainly increase. This is a good development and indicates that you are not reabsorbing toxins in your intestine. A mucous-coated stool will indicate that you are actually detoxing from the colon as well. Two to three bowel movements a day would be a very healthy number on this detox diet.

## Other symptoms

Detoxification can also induce nausea, aches and pains, fatigue and nasal discharge. This is because toxins are being released into the bloodstream at a faster rate than the liver can detoxify them. These symptoms will pass after a couple of days.

The best remedy is to go for a sauna or use a steam room. This forces the toxins out of the bloodstream and into the skin where they are released as sweat, bypassing the log-jammed liver. The best regimen is to sweat for 10–15 minutes, then to have a cold shower, then back into the sauna or steam room. Keep this up for as long as you feel comfortable but stop if you feel at all faint or dizzy. Drink even more water, as you will be losing a lot in sweat. If you can't cope with the heat, then go for a run to work up a sweat.

Eating some of the foods we have listed in this chapter may be new to you, but when you look through the collection of tasty liver-detox recipes that Fiona has prepared for you in the following chapter we are sure you will feel motivated and enthusiastic about getting started on your 9-Day Liver Detox. She also explains how to prepare our basic superfoods: the Essential Seed Mix and Super Greens Mix.

# CHAPTER **SIX**

# Your 9-Day Liver-detox Recipes

I feel particularly qualified to write the recipes for this book not only because I am a nutritionist and cook but also because I have recently undergone a detox myself. People always expect nutritionists to be positively radiating good health and vitality, but often the very reason that we turned to nutrition in the first place is because of our own health problems. I followed the detox rules here in order to sort out some skin problems while I was developing these recipes, and am happy to report great results! This has given me first-hand experience of what it is like to cut out favourite foods, not to mention an insight into the need for appetising recipes to boost morale when you are not feeling your best or are craving 'off limits' foods. The result, I hope, is a collection of recipes that are appetising and interesting and are positively packed with nutrients to cleanse your liver and boost your health.

There is no doubt about it, detoxing is hard work. It is hard work for your body, as your liver will be straining to keep up with pressure to eliminate waste and toxins, and it is hard work physically for you: mealtimes need planning and preparation. You cannot simply grab a sandwich or a plate of pasta, or boost flagging energy levels with a cup of coffee. We do understand that what we are asking you to do is hard, so we have taken particular care to come up with appetising, filling meals that should help to keep your spirits high during the nine-day plan.

*Fiona McDonald Joyce*

# Breakfast

It is important to start the day with a nutritious meal to kick-start your metabolism and provide you with energy at the best of times, but particularly so during a detox. Your liver function peaks between 2 am and 4 am so by the time you wake your body has already been at work for hours. You therefore need to refuel, and in particular get some protein inside you to allow the liver's detoxification process to continue. For those people who 'don't do breakfast' a smoothie or fresh juice is a refreshing and energising start to the day. You may also wish to have a glass of hot water with the juice of half a lemon freshly squeezed before eating in the morning. Lemons are very rich in vitamin C – much more so than their more acclaimed cousin the orange – and make a very cleansing drink to prepare your body for digestion and detoxification. You can add a couple of slices of fresh root ginger to the mug for a more warming flavour if you like.

## Why add the Essential Seed Mix?

Seeds are a vital part of your diet and are particularly helpful during a detox. They contain essential fats to keep your hormones in balance and your skin looking great, as well as minerals such as zinc to keep your immune system functioning and your blood sugar under control, and magnesium to give your thyroid a boost. They also provide protein, which your liver needs each day to detox efficiently and prevent the toxins you are releasing from being reabsorbed by the body. Our Essential Seed Mix is an easy way to include the recommended tablespoon of seeds in your diet at breakfast each day. Simply add a tablespoon of the ground seed mix to breakfast cereal, fruit salad or smoothies.

# The Essential Seed Mix

1 Half-fill a glass jar that has a sealing lid with flax seeds (also known as linseeds and rich in omega-3) and half with a mixture of sesame, sunflower and pumpkin seeds (rich in omega-6).

2 Keep the jar sealed and in the fridge to minimise damage from light, heat and oxygen.

3 Put a handful of the seed mix in a coffee or seed grinder (see Detox Tip overleaf), grind up and add a tablespoon to your cereal. Store the remainder in the fridge and use over the next few days.

4 To save time you could grind up to a week's worth of seeds, but make sure you store them away from heat, light and air to prevent the delicate essential fats from oxidising.

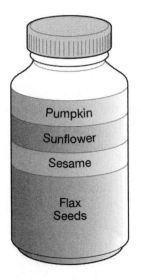

**The proportions of seeds in the Essential Seed Mix**

> ### DETOX TIP
>
> Grinding the seeds makes the nutrients in them available to the body, otherwise tiny seeds like flax seeds or sesame seeds are too small to be digested. If you don't have time to grind seeds you could simply sprinkle larger seeds such as pumpkin and sunflower seeds straight onto your food, together with pre-cracked or ground flax seeds, which you can buy from supermarkets (in the healthy-eating aisle) and health-food stores. Buy ones stored in foil or other light-proof packaging, however, to ensure that the fats are protected from oxidation before you can get them home and into the fridge.

Please note:

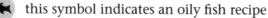

 this symbol indicates an oily fish recipe

✱ this symbol means the recipe is suitable for freezing

# Superfood Muesli

This thick, soaked muesli is delicious and particularly nutritious, as all the ingredients are raw, maximising the vitamin, enzyme and antioxidant content. Apples contain the phyto-nutrient quercetin, which is a natural anti-inflammatory to help allergies, asthma, eczema and arthritis. Oats are a fibre-rich, low Glycemic Load (GL) carbohydrate; that is, they release their energy very slowly to keep you feeling fuller for longer; they also contain the amino acid tryptophan, which the brain converts into the 'feel good' neurotransmitter serotonin.

**SERVES 1**

40g (1½oz) whole rolled porridge oats

1 tbsp ground almonds or desiccated coconut

1 tbsp Essential Seed Mix (see page 109)

½ small apple, grated

1 tbsp berries, such as raspberries or blueberries

½ tsp ground cinnamon, or to taste (optional)

Place all the ingredients in a bowl and cover with double the amount of boiling water. Stir and leave to thicken for a couple of minutes until the oats have soaked up the water and become soft and plump.

# Cinnamon Fruit Porridge

Oats are full of soluble fibre for healthy digestion and release their energy very slowly to keep you filled up. Cinnamon not only adds a wonderfully warming flavour but it is also a valuable nutrient, helping the body regulate blood-sugar levels. Ground ginger can be used instead of the cinnamon or as well, if you prefer.

**SERVES 1**

40g (1½oz) whole rolled porridge oats

½–1 tsp ground cinnamon, or to taste

1 tbsp Essential Seed Mix (see page 109)

plus any fruit, chopped, grated, or left whole if berries
   (see Cook's Tip below)

1 Place the oats in a pan and cover with water. Bring to the boil then gently simmer, stirring, until the porridge thickens and the oats soften.

2 Stir the cinnamon, seed mix and fruit into the porridge, or simply scatter on top of the porridge in a bowl.

## COOK'S TIP

Chop or grate ½ an apple, or chop up a pear or a couple of plums or apricots, or simply toss some berries into the porridge and let them soften in the heat so that they burst and release their sweet juice.

# Toast and Nut Butter

■

Here we use pumpernickel-style rye bread, as it contains less gluten than wheat, making it much easier to digest. Plus, whole-grain rye is a good source of prebiotics, feeding the good bacteria in your gut. Spread it with nut or seed butter (you can get a whole range of different nut and seed butters in health-food stores) to add some protein to help fuel your liver's detoxification pathways, as well as filling you up.

**SERVES 1**

1 thin slice pumpernickel-style rye bread

1 tbsp (or enough to spread on each slice) nut or seed butter
   (almond and hazelnut are particularly good)

Toast the bread then spread the butter straight on to each slice. There is enough natural oil in nuts and seeds for you not to miss the absence of normal butter – honestly.

# Super-fruit and Seed Salad

■

If going on a detox makes you feel instantly deprived as you give up your usual morning cappuccino or croissant, think about the money you will be saving and splash out instead on some tropical fruit or fresh berries to enliven breakfast. The bright, vibrant colours not only look wonderful but they are also packed with phyto-nutrients like flavonoids, to really kick-start your immune system. Apply the Rainbow Rule opposite and try to get as many different colours into your bowl as possible, as each colour indicates a different type of plant nutrient.

**SERVES 1**

the seeds of ½ pomegranate

watermelon chunks (leave the seeds in as they are rich in vitamin E)

a couple of handfuls of blueberries

OR

mango slices

banana slices

strawberries

sliced kiwi fruit

a good squeeze of fresh lemon juice

1 tbsp of Essential Seed Mix (see page 109)

Mix the fruits in a bowl with the seed mix and add the lemon juice. (Lemon juice not only adds a pleasing tartness to complement the sweet fruit but also the vitamin C prevents the cut fruit from oxidising and going brown and the liquid helps loosen the texture of the dry seeds.)

## THE RAINBOW RULE

Aim to eat as many different-coloured fruits and vegetables as possible, as each colour denotes a particular health benefit. For example, yellow and orange plants such as squash, peppers and sweet potatoes are rich in the antioxidant vitamin beta-carotene, which has valuable anti-ageing properties, whereas the rich pinks, purples and blues in berries are high in free-radical-scavenging flavonoids, which again will help you hold back the years. In your super-fruit salad try unpeeled apples, pears, greengages, apricots, peaches, nectarines, plums, oranges, tangerines, kiwi or pomegranate to vary the colours. By eating the fruit raw you benefit from all of the nutrient content; from the vitamins and minerals to phytonutrients and enzymes. Plus, fruit is packed with fibre and water, both of which will keep your digestive system working and help reduce bloating.

# Berry Breakfast Smoothie

■

If you don't have the time or inclination for breakfast, then go for a smoothie. You can drink it on the run and it is packed with all the nutrients you need: carbohydrate, vitamins and minerals from the fruit and essential fats and protein from the seeds. This can count as your breakfast or as your daily smoothie (according to our Six Golden Liver-detox Rules on page 102), but not as both. Blueberries are particularly rich in immune and liver-boosting flavonoids but you can vary the fruit used. Also, after your detox when you can eat dairy products again, try thickening the smoothie with live, natural yoghurt to add extra protein and beneficial probiotic bacteria.

### SERVES 1

1 small banana, or ½ medium one, not too ripe

2 teaspoons Essential Seed Mix (see page 109)

1 small punnet, 150g (5½oz), blueberries or other berries

juice of ½ lemon

plus enough pure fruit juice (orange works well) or unsweetened
   rice milk (or other non-dairy milk, see Detox Tip below) or water
   to give an easy-to-drink consistency (or leave thick and eat with a
   spoon)

Blend all the ingredients together until smooth.

> **DETOX TIP**
>
> Other non-dairy milks to try are quinoa, almond, oat, soya or coconut milk.

# Snacks

Here are some quick snack ideas to keep your energy levels balanced and your liver functioning efficiently. They are all super-quick to make and there are lots of easy, convenient options such as fruit and nuts to keep in your drawer at work or in your bag if you are out and about.

## Fruit

It's not original, but fruit is about as fast as food gets and, of course, it is incredibly good for you. Again, think beyond the usual apple or orange (although these are still nutrient-packed choices) to get some different colours and phytonutrients into your diet. You could pick at a punnet of berries, or have fresh apricots, a slice of melon or a pink grapefruit, or perhaps kiwi, mango or red grapes rather than green. If you are the kind of person who normally peels their apple or pear, don't – much of the goodness is stored in the skin and seeds of fruit, and you will find that eating a whole pear instead of stopping at the core is perfectly palatable. The same goes for grapes – go for seeded rather than the more expensive seedless varieties – and for watermelon – the seeds are rich in the skin-friendly antioxidant vitamin E.

Have a small handful (around a tablespoon) of nuts or seeds with your fruit to provide extra protein, which will fill you up for longer and boost the detoxification process.

## Nuts and seeds

Pick on a small handful (around a tablespoon) of unsalted, unroasted nuts or seeds (such as pecan nuts, almonds, walnuts, Brazil nuts, hazelnuts, pumpkin seeds or sunflower seeds, or a mixture of your favourites). Eating nuts or seeds with fruit helps to keep blood sugar even, as the protein slows down the sugar released from the fruit. They are also packed with minerals such as zinc, which is involved in everything from your immune system to hormone balance and even libido.

# Roasted Pumpkin Seeds

◼

Heat up a frying pan before putting the pumpkin seeds into it (no oil needed) and cook for a couple of minutes, tossing the seeds in the pan occasionally, until they start to pop and go golden.

## Olives

Olives contain the heart-helping monounsaturated fats. They are also a quick and easy snack that is very more-ish. Look out for ones stuffed with whole garlic cloves or almonds, for extra liver-boosting power. Eat a couple of handfuls, or about 8 olives as a snack.

## Avocado

Rich in heart-friendly monounsaturated fats, avocados also contain vitamin E. Avocados act as 'nutrient boosters', increasing the body's ability to absorb fat-soluble nutrients like alpha- and beta-carotene from other foods. They also provide over 25 nutrients, including fibre, potassium, vitamin E, B vitamins, and folic acid. A couple over the course of the nine-day plan are fine but don't have too many, as you don't want to add too much fat to your diet. A half or a whole avocado makes a delicious snack: simply cut in half, remove the stone and drizzle with lemon juice or enjoy it plain. You can also follow the Mexicans' example and mash avocado on to toast or oat-cakes instead of butter. If you are eating only half, keep the stone in the remaining half, drizzle with lemon juice, wrap in cling-film and keep in the fridge to prevent it from discolouring. Eat it the next day.

## Hummus with Crudités

Hummus is a brilliant snack and light-meal standby for when you are busy. The chickpeas in hummus provide protein plus fibre and phytoestrogens to help keep your hormones in balance, while the garlic will top up your sulphur levels to help your liver's detoxification capacity. Grab a pot from the chiller aisle in the supermarket or deli and dip in crudités such as celery, apple, cucumber and pepper strips, or oatcakes for a more substantial snack or light lunch. Shop-bought hummus will contain a little salt, but it still makes a healthy and extremely convenient choice during a detox, and makes for a perfect detox snack or lunch on the go. Stir in a dollop of the Super Greens Mix (see page 122) to make it extra healthy.

# Guacamole

■

If you have a little more time you can make this delicious, very refreshing avocado dip and serve it with crudités. Don't just stick to the usual carrot, celery and cucumber crudités; try sugar snap peas, baby corn, white cabbage, radishes, spring onions, celeriac, peppers, cherry tomatoes and fennel.

**SERVES 2**

1 ripe avocado

juice of ¼ lemon

½ garlic clove, crushed

¼ small red onion, finely diced

3 cherry tomatoes, finely diced

1 tbsp chopped fresh coriander and/or flat-leaf parsley (optional)

1 tbsp extra virgin olive oil, or omega-rich seed oil like flax seed
    (linseed), hemp or pumpkin seed oil (optional)

freshly ground black pepper

1 Cut the avocado in half lengthways and remove the stone.

2 Scrape the flesh out of the shell into a bowl and quickly mash with the remaining ingredients then taste to check the seasoning. (Keep any leftovers covered in the fridge for up to two days.)

# Corn on the Cob

■

This is a very filling snack and the bright yellow corn kernels are packed with beta-carotene, an essential antioxidant for the skin. Most people slather corn on the cob in butter but corn has so much natural sweetness and juiciness that you honestly don't need anything on it other than perhaps a splash of lemon juice. This makes a really healthy snack but you can also slice off the corn kernels and scatter on salads, soups or stir-fries.

**SERVES 1**

1 corn on the cob

1 Cut off the stalk end of the cob and peel away the outer husk and silk. Trim off the pointed end. Place a couple of sheets of kitchen paper on a large plate.

2 Bring a pan of water to the boil then place the cob in the pan and boil for between 5–15 minutes (until a kernel of corn comes away easily). Don't add salt to the pan – it is not only off the menu during the nine-day plan but will also toughen the corn.

3 Remove from the pan and place the cob on the kitchen paper to absorb any excess moisture. You can drizzle with lemon juice if you like. Eat with your fingers or use corn skewers.

# Main meals

These main meals have been split into Cold Meals and Hot Meals. The Cold Meals (see page 124) contain salads, sandwiches, dips and even a raw soup, which make quick and easy lunches, and the Hot Meals (see page 131) include soups and stews, so that you can look forward to a warming, filling supper at the end of the day. These are flexible, however, so if the weather is warm and you feel like having salad for lunch and for supper, then do. Equally, if you want something hot at both meals, then have soup for lunch and stew for supper. The one rule we do insist on is that you have the Super Greens Mix (see below) with at least one main meal each day. This blend of super-greens such as parsley, basil, watercress and baby spinach is a great way to eat far more leaves and herbs than you normally would in a simple salad and will give your liver a huge boost. It also adds colour and flavour to soups and stews.

 this symbol indicates an oily fish recipe

✱ this symbol means the recipe is suitable for freezing

## Super Greens Mix

This pesto-style blend of dark green leaves and herbs is a brilliant way to increase your intake dramatically of these flavonoid and vitamin-C rich ingredients without having to wade through buckets of salad. Simply blend it all together with some oil and lemon juice and serve on soups, salads and main meals. We recommend you have a serving of this on at least one of your meals each day, ideally two, to give your liver a helping hand. You can vary the leaves and herbs used according to taste and availability. Add avocado (rich in vitamin E and protein) for a thicker consistency, or cucumber (a very cleansing vegetable) for a thinner texture. Equally, you can ring the changes by adding raw garlic (to get your daily intake of sulphurous vegetables), sun-blush tomatoes or roasted peppers, olives, marinated artichoke hearts, pumpkin seeds or pine nuts.

### SERVES 1

¼ bag (a good handful) watercress, rinsed and dried

¼ bag (a good handful) baby leaf spinach, rinsed and dried

a good handful of basil leaves

a good handful of parsley leaves

a good drizzle, about 1tbsp, of extra virgin olive oil or an omega-rich
     seed oil such as hemp or flax seed oil

squeeze of lemon juice, to taste

Whizz all the ingredients together in a mini blender or food processor, or, if you don't have one of these handy, finely chop the herbs. Stir in the oil; the mixture should hold together a little like pesto.

> **DETOX TIP**
>
> Vegetarians and vegans who will not be eating the recommended two portions of oily fish in the nine-day plan should use the omega-rich seed oil like hemp or flaxseed oil, to ensure that they obtain omega-3 fats.

# Cold meals

These recipes can all be eaten cold so they make ideal packed lunches to take to work or grab from the fridge. Some do involve a little cooking beforehand, but they are all simple and quick to prepare. You can choose from open rye sandwiches, salads and even a raw soup, which is perfect for summer.

## Superboost Sesame Salad

■

The strong flavours of toasted sesame oil and lemon juice breathe life into this easy-to-make salad without adding any salt or spices. Celery is rich in the mineral potassium, which helps to lower blood pressure, while the chickpeas provide phytoestrogens to help balance hormones, which in turn reduces strain on your liver to regulate levels.

**SERVES 2** (or double the quantities for a more substantial meal)

1 × 410g (14½oz) can chickpeas, rinsed and drained

2 celery sticks, finely chopped

6 pieces marinated artichoke heart, roughly chopped

6 spring onions, finely chopped

1 tbsp sesame seeds (untoasted)

1 tsp toasted sesame oil, or to taste

juice of ½ a lemon

Mix all of the ingredients together and serve with salad, including a portion of Super Greens Mix (see page 122) if you like.

# Superfood Sandwich for Beautiful Skin

■

The salmon in this sandwich provides one of your recommended three servings of omega-3 essential fats during the nine-day plan. Both salmon and watercress are also excellent sources of zinc, which both men and women need for a healthy libido. What's more, watercress contains greater quantities of the antioxidant carotenoids lutein and zeaxanthin as well as vitamin C than apples and broccoli, to help mop up damaging free radicals. All in all this truly is a superfood sandwich.

### SERVES 1

1 salmon fillet (preferably organic)
½ portion Super Greens Mix (see page 122)
1 large (or 2 small) slices pumpernickel-style rye bread (choose a
    yeast-free brand)
squeeze of lemon juice

1 Steam the salmon fillet for about 15 minutes, or until cooked (it should flake easily when pressed). Skin and flake (checking for bones as you do so) and allow it to cool.

2 Spread the greens mix on toasted (or untoasted if you prefer) rye bread and top with the flaked salmon and a squeeze of lemon juice.

**DETOX TIP**

In your Super Greens Mix do use watercress, as the peppery flavour is the perfect partner for salmon. Make sure you use enough oil to give this a pesto-type consistency for ease of spreading.

# Skin-defence Dip

■

The aubergine and borlotti beans in this dip give a smoky, rich flavour to this delicious blend of vegetables. Cooked tomato products, such as tomato purée, are a better source of lycopene than raw tomatoes. This antioxidant nutrient not only helps to protect eyesight but it has also been shown to reduce skin damage by UV rays by as much as 30 per cent! Consider it an edible sunscreen to keep wrinkles at bay. Serve this dip with crudités and oatcakes or spread on pumpernickel-style rye bread and top with watercress, rocket or baby spinach.

**SERVES 2**

1 tsp coconut oil or medium (not extra virgin) olive oil

1 garlic clove, crushed

1 red onion, diced

¼ medium aubergine, cubed

1 tbsp tomato purée

½ × 410g can borlotti beans, rinsed and drained

1 tsp Marigold Reduced Salt Vegetable Bouillon powder

2 portions of Super Greens Mix (see page 122)

1 Heat the oil and sauté the garlic and onion for a couple of minutes to let the onion start to soften then throw in the aubergine and cook for a few minutes until it browns and softens.

2 Add the tomato purée, beans and bouillon powder, and stir together.

3 Place the mixture in a food processor or blender and whizz until fairly smooth. You can also add Super Greens Mix to the mixture to blend at the same time, if you like, or stir in afterwards.

# Cleansing Bean and Artichoke Salad

This dish is surprisingly filling and full-flavoured, and is equally good served hot or cold. It is rich in the detox mineral sulphur, from the garlic and onions, as well as being packed with digestion-boosting fibre, including inulin in the artichokes, which encourages beneficial probiotic bacteria to flourish in the gut.

## SERVES 2

2 garlic cloves, crushed

1 red onion, finely diced

1 tbsp coconut oil or 2 tbsp medium (not extra virgin) olive oil

250g (9oz) cherry tomatoes, chopped

2 tbsp tomato purée

1 × 410g can mixed pulses, drained and rinsed

6 marinated artichoke heart halves from a jar or the deli, roughly
   chopped

2 tbsp black olives, pitted and roughly chopped (optional)

handful of fresh basil leaves, torn – or a dollop of Super Greens Mix
   (see page 122)

1  Sweat the garlic and onion in the oil in a frying pan for about 3 minutes until translucent.

2  Add the tomatoes and cook for a couple of minutes until they disintegrate.

3  Stir in the tomato purée, mixed pulses, artichoke hearts and olives, reduce the heat and simmer for about 5 minutes or until thick and rich – you can add a splash of water to loosen it if the sauce dries up. Add the basil or Super Greens Mix just before serving.

# Superfood Salad of Quinoa with Roasted Veg

■

Research has shown that consuming vitamin E and the nutrient lycopene together, such as in the pumpkin seeds and tomatoes used here, enhances their positive antioxidant effects. Surprisingly, the antioxidant lycopene in tomatoes is more readily absorbed by the body when the tomatoes are cooked, so these roasted cherry tomatoes are ideal. Regular consumption of lycopene has been shown to reduce the skin's damage from ultraviolet rays from the sun. This, combined with the zinc and protein-rich quinoa and the liver-boosting herbs, makes a superfood meal. Make this meal in advance and eat it cold or warm, but it is also delicious hot, either on its own or with rocket. Add some fresh lemon juice for a zesty flavour, if you like.

### SERVES 2

1 small sweet potato, skin left on, cubed

1 small red onion, roughly chopped

1 red, yellow or orange pepper, roughly chopped

1 small courgette, roughly chopped

2 garlic cloves, thinly sliced

drizzle (about 1–2 tbsp) medium (not extra virgin) olive oil

200g (7oz) cherry tomatoes

150g (5½oz) quinoa

1 tsp Marigold Reduced Salt Vegetable Bouillon powder

2 heaped tbsp pumpkin seeds

2 portions Super Greens Mix (see page 122)

1 Preheat the oven to 200°C/400°F/Gas 6. Place the chopped vegetables and garlic in a roasting tin, drizzle with oil, stir to coat then cook for 40 minutes. Add the whole cherry tomatoes and return

to the oven for a further 15–20 minutes, until the tomato skins split and the sweet potatoes are soft when pierced.

2 Meanwhile, place the quinoa and bouillon powder in a pan and cover with boiling water (two parts water to one part quinoa). Bring to the boil then cover, reduce the heat and simmer for about 12–15 minutes until the liquid is absorbed and the grains are fluffy. Set to one side, covered, while the vegetables finish cooking.

3 Five minutes before the vegetables are ready, place the pumpkin seeds on a baking tray and pop them in the oven on the top shelf to toast.

4 Stir the roasted vegetables and the Super Greens Mix into the quinoa then sprinkle the toasted pumpkin seeds on top. Leave to cool or eat warm, if you prefer.

# Raw Summer Soup

■

This soup maximises the nutrient content of its ingredients, as they are served raw. Cucumber and lemons are both very cleansing for the liver, whereas the avocado and olive oil provide heart-friendly monounsaturated fat. Avocados are also rich in vitamin E, which helps to keep your skin in good condition.

### SERVES 2

1 avocado, stoned and the flesh scooped out of the skin
½ cucumber, roughly chopped
175g (6oz) cherry tomatoes
small handful of fresh basil leaves
2 tbsp cold pressed oil (extra virgin olive oil or flax seed or hemp oil)
juice of ¼ lemon

**FOR THE GARNISH**
2 spring onions, finely sliced on the diagonal
OR
2 portions of Super Greens Mix (see page 122)

Blend all the ingredients until smooth then pour into bowls and sprinkle with spring onions or spoon on the greens mix to garnish. Eat immediately or chill until ready to serve.

# Hot meals

Here are some warming, filling recipes for comfort food during your detox. There is no need to go hungry when you are avoiding foods like meat, dairy products and refined grains – we have included masses of fresh, wholesome ingredients to help nourish you back to health. These are intended as suppers or main meals, when you have a little more time, but equally the stews and soups could be eaten for lunch. You could take some to work in a vacuum flask or reheat a portion.

## Baked Sweet Potatoes with Borlotti Stew

Sweet potatoes are incredibly rich in antioxidant vitamins beta-carotene and vitamin E, both of which are required to keep the immune system functioning and to keep skin in good condition. They are deliciously smooth and sweet when baked, and make a very filling, warming meal when topped with this rich, thick ragout-style bean stew.

**SERVES 2**

2 large sweet potatoes
a little medium (not extra virgin) olive oil

**FOR THE STEW**

1 tbsp coconut oil or olive oil
2 garlic cloves, crushed
1 large red onion, diced
100g (4oz) mushrooms, sliced (see Cook's Tip overleaf)
2 tbsp tomato purée
1 × 400g can plum tomatoes
1 × 410g can borlotti beans, drained and rinsed
½ tsp Marigold Reduced Salt Vegetable Bouillon powder
½ tsp herbes de Provence, or to taste
freshly ground black pepper

1 Preheat the oven to 200°C/400°F/Gas 6. Prick the potatoes all over. Rub with a little oil and place on a baking tray. Cook for 1 hour, or until soft all the way through when pierced with a knife.

2 Meanwhile, prepare the stew. Heat the oil in a pan and sweat the garlic and onion gently for 2 minutes, then add the mushrooms and cook for 5 minutes, or until fairly soft.

3 Add the remaining ingredients and simmer for about 5–10 minutes to allow the vegetables to soften and the sauce to thicken. Check the seasoning and adjust if necessary.

4 Open up the baked potatoes and spoon the stew inside.

**COOK'S TIP**

To clean mushrooms, wipe with a soft brush or a piece of kitchen paper.

# Patrick's Primordial Soup

■

This soup was designed by Patrick to help his wife Gaby get over a virus and it's now highly regarded as a renowned health tonic by his readers! It is so-called because it contains foods that provide the key nutrients to ensure good health. It is incredibly rich in vitamin E and beta-carotene, as well as anti-inflammatory onions, garlic and ginger. The coconut milk not only gives a rich, creamy flavour, it also contains medium-chain triglycerides – special kinds of saturated fat that are not stored as fat but are used to give you energy. Coconut is also thought to help thyroid function and to fight infection.

## SERVES 2–3

1 tbsp coconut oil or medium (not extra virgin) olive oil

½ red onion, roughly chopped

1 garlic clove, crushed

1 large carrot or 2 small–medium ones, peeled and chopped

1 large sweet potato, or 2 small–medium ones, not peeled, chopped
    to the same size as the carrot to ensure even cooking

1 heaped tsp grated fresh root ginger (see Cook's Tip on page 135)

¼ tsp turmeric

2 tsp Marigold Reduced Salt Vegetable Bouillon powder

½ red pepper, diced

75ml (2½fl oz) coconut milk

1   Heat the oil in a large pan and gently sauté the onion and garlic for a few minutes until they start to soften but do not turn brown.

2   Add the carrot, sweet potato, ginger, turmeric and bouillon powder. Just cover with boiling water and bring to the boil. Cover and simmer for about 15 minutes or until the vegetables are soft.

3   Add the red pepper and coconut milk, then blend until smooth and thick.

# Leek, Cannellini and Potato Soup

■

This is a slight twist on a classic that will fill you up and boost flagging energy levels. Leeks are a good source of prebiotics, which provide fuel for the digestion and immune system to boost probiotic bacteria. They also, along with the garlic, provide sulphur to assist your liver's detox capacity. We have added high fibre, low-GL cannellini beans to help thicken the soup and create a creamy consistency.

### SERVES 2 ✱

1 tsp coconut oil or olive oil

2 cloves garlic, crushed

2 large leeks (300g/11oz trimmed weight), trimmed and well rinsed, then sliced

2 medium or 3 small baby new potatoes (approximately 75g/3oz), unpeeled and cubed

600ml (1pt) boiling water

3 tsp Marigold Reduced Salt Vegetable Bouillon powder

1 x 410g can cannellini beans, rinsed and drained

Freshly ground black pepper

2 servings of Super Greens Mix (if required for daily serving)

1 Heat the oil in a pan and sauté the garlic for 30 seconds.

2 Add the leeks, cover and sweat for 3 minutes until they start to soften.

3 Tip the potatoes, water and bouillon powder into the pan and stir then cover and simmer for 15 minutes.

4 Add the beans and blend with a handheld blender until fairly smooth. Season with black pepper then add a dollop of Super Greens Mix (see page 122), if using.

### COOK'S TIP

Beans are a better source of carbohydrate than potatoes for anyone with blood sugar imbalances, such as diabetics, or for sugar addicts. As they are digested slowly they cause a gradual rise in blood sugar in contrast to the rapid but short-lived burst of energy from potatoes. Beans are also recommended for clearing arteries, in part because of their choline content, which is used for fat metabolism. Their high-fibre content makes beans excellent for preventing constipation and improving stool transit time.

# Age-defying Carrot and Lentil Soup

■

Thick and filling, this soup is perfect to keep in the fridge ready for an instant meal. The bright orange colour shows how rich this soup is in the antioxidant vitamin beta-carotene, which will mop up free radicals to prevent them from damaging cells. Lentils also provide more folic acid than any other unfortified food. Folic acid is not only important for pregnant women, it is also a vital nutrient for everyone, as it helps reduce your risk of age-related degenerative diseases.

**SERVES 4** ✱

1 tbsp coconut oil, olive oil or butter

2 garlic cloves, crushed

1 onion, roughly chopped

2 large celery sticks, sliced

4 medium-large carrots, sliced

200g (7oz) red split lentils, rinsed

1 litre (1¾ pints) hot vegetable stock (see Cook's Tip below)

1 Heat the oil in a large pan and sweat the garlic and onion for 5 minutes to soften.

2 Add the celery, carrots, lentils and stock, then stir and bring to the boil. Cover and simmer for 10 minutes to allow the carrots to soften, then blend until smooth or your preferred consistency.

## COOK'S TIP

For a quick stock, we like 1 litre (1¾ pints) boiling water mixed with 2–3 tsp Marigold Reduced Salt Vegetable Bouillon powder, to make 8 ladlefuls. Freeze or chill any leftovers.

# Fennel and Mixed Rice Pilaff

■

This dish has a subtle mixture of flavours and textures, from the soft, slightly sweet fennel and onions to the crunchy wild rice. Fennel is an excellent liver booster and the wild rice (which is actually a grass) provides more protein and minerals than standard rice. The recipe is delicious cold (you can eat this for supper and then take some to work the next day for lunch).

### SERVES 2 ✱

1 tsp Marigold Reduced Salt Vegetable Bouillon powder

90g (3¼oz) mixed rice (wild rice, brown basmati rice and red Camargue rice) (see Cook's Tip overleaf)

1 tbsp coconut oil or olive oil

1 small or ½ large red onion, peeled and cut into thin wedges

½ fennel bulb, thinly sliced lengthways

115g (4½oz) chestnut mushrooms, quartered

½ × 410g can green lentils, drained and rinsed

1 tbsp lemon juice

2 tbsp finely chopped flat-leaf parsley

freshly ground black pepper

1 Bring a large pan of water to the boil and add the bouillon powder. Cook the rice according to the pack instructions. As the grains are unrefined they should be tender when cooked but will still retain some bite. Drain the rice.

2 While the rice is cooking, heat the oil in a medium–large frying pan and cook the onion, fennel and mushrooms over a medium–high heat for 5–10 minutes, until they soften. Reduce the heat while you prepare the rice.

3 Add the rice to the pan of vegetables along with the lentils, and stir over a low–medium heat. Add the lemon juice, parsley and lots of black pepper. Taste to check the seasoning before serving. Serve with a mixed leaf salad.

## COOK'S TIP

You can buy mixed rice ready-mixed from health-food stores, or you could make up your own combination.

# Rice with Super-greens Pesto

■

A cross between a pesto and a tapenade, the combination of olives and herbs in the sauce for this dish adds flavour and texture as well as topping up your nutrient levels, of course. The pumpkin seeds provide protein and zinc, while the olives are not only a good source of heart-friendly monounsaturated fats but they are also rich in vitamin E as well as flavonoids, both of which appear to have anti-inflammatory properties. Serve warm or cold with a large mixed salad that includes some tomato and thinly sliced red onion for colour. If you have more time, griddled or grilled courgettes make an attractive and delicious accompaniment: thinly slice them lengthways and marinate for ten minutes in a little lemon juice and olive oil before lightly griddling or grilling for 30 seconds or so.

**SERVES 2**

150g (5½oz) brown basmati rice, rinsed

**FOR THE SUPER-GREENS PESTO**
2 portions of Super Greens Mix (see page 122)
2 tbsp pumpkin seeds, lightly toasted for a couple of minutes in a
     dry frying pan until they start to swell and 'pop'
6 tbsp pitted Kalamata olives
2 tbsp extra virgin olive oil (from the jar if the olives are stored in oil)
2 large garlic cloves crushed
4 handfuls of fresh basil leaves
2 handfuls of rocket
2 handfuls of baby spinach or flat-leaf parsley leaves
freshly ground black pepper
juice of a lemon, or to taste

1 Cook the rice according to the instructions on the packet (about 20 minutes).

2 Meanwhile, prepare the super-greens pesto. Whizz all the ingredients together in a mini blender or food processor. Taste to check the flavour – you can add more of any of the ingredients to tweak the flavour, if you like. Toss the pesto through the rice. Serve warm with a large mixed salad.

# Mushroom and Pine Nut Stuffed Peppers

■

Peppers are very high in antioxidants and vitamin C. They are delicious served here stuffed with a rich rice mixture of pine nuts, basil and mushrooms. To make this even healthier, choose shiitake mushrooms for their lentinan content, as this polysaccharide is a powerful immune booster long used in Traditional Chinese Medicine.

**SERVES 2**

2 large red peppers
1 tbsp coconut oil or olive oil
1 medium onion, finely chopped
2 garlic cloves, crushed
150g (5½oz) mushrooms, sliced
1 tsp Marigold Reduced Salt Vegetable Bouillon powder
115g (4½oz) brown basmati rice, cooked, 50g (2oz) raw weight
1 tbsp nuts (see Cook's Tip opposite)
handful of fresh basil, chopped

1 Preheat the oven to 200°C/400°F/Gas 6. Cut the tops off the peppers (reserving them to make lids) and remove the seeds and pith.

2 Heat the oil in a sauté pan and gently fry the onion and garlic for 2 minutes. Add the chopped mushrooms and bouillon powder and fry for a further 2–3 minutes.

3 Transfer to a large bowl and add the cooked rice, nuts and basil.

4 Stuff the peppers with the mixture and place the tops back on.

5 Place on a baking tray and bake for 35 minutes.

**COOK'S TIP**

Pine nuts taste wonderful in this dish, but they are expensive. Cheaper alternatives include chopped walnuts or cashew nuts, or flaked almonds. Or use sunflower or pumpkin seeds for a nut-free version.

# Trout en Papillote with Roasted Vegetables

◾

Cooking fish *en papillote* (in a parcel of baking parchment) preserves all of its juices, flavour and essential fats. This recipe is bursting with colour, from the orange-fleshed sweet potatoes to the vibrant green of the greens mix, all of which contribute to its high antioxidant content. The garlic, parsley and lemon juice all provide flavour as well as nutrients – garlic is rich in sulphur and is a powerful anti-inflammatory, whereas parsley and lemons are rich in vitamin C.

**SERVES 2**

2 medium or 1 large sweet potato, sliced into fairly thin wedges

2 courgettes, sliced into similar-sized wedges

drizzle (about 1 tbsp) of mild (not extra virgin) olive oil

2 medium-sized rainbow trout (preferably organic), fully prepared

2 garlic cloves, crushed

juice of 1 lemon

2 teaspoons fresh flat-leaf parsley leaves, finely chopped

2 portions of Super Greens Mix (see page 122)

1 Preheat the oven to 180°C/350°F/Gas 4. Place the sweet potatoes and courgettes in a roasting tin, drizzle with the oil and roast for about 1 hour, stirring to turn the vegetables over halfway through, until the sweet potatoes are soft when pierced with a knife.

2 Meanwhile, take a large piece of baking parchment, large enough to cover both fish lying diagonally across the middle of the paper when folded in half on the diagonal.

3 Season the inside of each fish with the garlic, lemon juice and parsley, and place the fish diagonally across the baking paper then fold in half on the diagonal.

4 Starting from one end, gradually fold up the edges to seal the paper into a parcel, overlapping each fold slightly over the last fold to stop it unravelling.

5 Place the parcel on a baking tray and bake for 25 minutes. Unwrap carefully to avoid being burned by the steam, and place the fish on plates with the cooked vegetables and a portion of Super Greens Mix each. Serve immediately.

## COOK'S TIP

The reason why we suggest you bake the fish in baking paper rather than kitchen foil is that the aluminium in kitchen foil can leach into your food, particularly if it comes into contact with acidic ingredients such as the lemon juice in this recipe. Some evidence points to high aluminium levels being implicated in Alzheimer's disease.

# Salmon with Puy Lentils

■

Here is another omega-3-rich fish dish to keep your essential-fat levels up during the detox plan, as well as providing protein to fuel your liver's detoxification pathways and your body's repair work. Steaming the salmon helps to preserve as much of the valuable omega-3 fats as possible, because it is a much gentler cooking technique than the direct, fierce heat from a frying pan or grill. Puy lentils not only hold their shape when cooked, providing texture to the dish, but they are also very rich in protein, and are combined here with antioxidant-dense tomato purée and sulphur-rich leeks to create a filling and nutritious stew to serve with the salmon. The dish is also delicious cold.

**SERVES 2**

115g (4½oz) Puy lentils, well rinsed

2 tsp Marigold Reduced Salt Vegetable Bouillon powder

2 leeks, finely sliced

2 salmon fillets (preferably organic)

2 tbsp tomato purée

splash of water

squeeze of fresh lemon juice

2 portions Super Greens Mix (see page 122)

freshly ground black pepper

1 Place the lentils in a pan and cover with double the amount of water. Add the bouillon powder. Bring to the boil then cover and simmer for 20–25 minutes until the lentils are al dente (firm to the bite), adding the leeks to the pan halfway through cooking. The lentils will absorb most of the liquid during cooking.

2 Put the salmon in a steamer pan and steam for about 15 minutes or until cooked – the flesh should flake easily when pressed. (Alternatively, if you don't have steamer, put the fish in a shallow pan,

cover with water and simmer gently until the flesh flakes when pressed.)

3 Stir the tomato purée into the lentil mixture along with a splash of water and squeeze of lemon to loosen the consistency and produce a thick stew.

4 Either serve the salmon on a bed of stew and scatter the Super Greens Mix over the top, or fold the greens mixture into the stew before topping with the fish. Sprinkle with freshly ground black pepper.

# Desserts

These desserts serve two purposes: firstly, to increase your fruit and antioxidant intake, and secondly, to keep your morale high during the nine-day detox plan when you are cutting out other foods. We recommend you have a pudding on each of the weekends, one at the start of the detox and the other at the end, to spread out your treats and give you something to look forward to, but it is entirely up to you when you include them. The recipes have not only passed testers' stringent taste tests but they are also a valuable source of vitamins, fibre and other plant nutrients, plus protein to enable your liver to detoxify efficiently.

## Fruit Burst Frozen Yoghurt

This pudding does contain dairy products, which are otherwise to be avoided on the nine-day detox, but the organic live natural yoghurt provides valuable probiotic bacteria, which will give your digestive and immune systems a boost. Probiotics populate the gut wall to prevent harmful bacteria from taking hold. The creamy yoghurt also helps to give the same smooth texture as a sorbet or ice cream. The berries are packed with vitamin C and bioflavonoids all of which will top up your body's own levels.

**SERVES 4**

400g (14oz) frozen mixed berries (available in bags from
   supermarkets)
400g (14oz) live natural yoghurt
4 tbsp xylitol (see page 147), or to taste

Blend all the ingredients together until smooth and the consistency of sorbet or frozen yoghurt. Eat quickly before it melts (although if it does melt it makes a delicious drink).

**COOK'S TIP**

Leave the frozen berries to defrost for a few minutes first if your blender won't cope with fully frozen ones.

# Detox Pear and Blueberry Crumble

■

A comfort-food pudding to cheer you up if you are going through sugar withdrawal symptoms. Standard crumbles are high in refined wheat, butter and sugar but our liver-friendly version replaces flour with oats and almonds, and is dairy and sugar free. It is rich in vitamins, minerals and fibre, to help digestion and detoxification. The addition of ginger not only adds a warming flavour but it is also a very effective, natural anti-inflammatory, whereas cinnamon helps improve glucose tolerance to balance blood-sugar levels.

**SERVES 2**

2 medium or large pears, cored and roughly chopped

a small punnet, about 150g (5½oz) of blueberries

splash of water

ground ginger and/or cinnamon, to taste

**FOR THE CRUMBLE**

2 tbsp coconut oil or medium (not extra virgin) olive oil

1 tbsp xylitol (naturally occurring sugar alternative which does not upset blood-sugar levels)

50g (2oz) whole oat flakes

2 heaped tbsp ground almonds

2 tbsp flaked almonds, or other roughly chopped nuts such as pecan nuts, hazelnuts, walnuts, or pumpkin seeds or sunflower seeds

1 Place the fruit in a pan with the water, cover, and stew gently for a about 5 minutes until the fruit softens, stirring from time to time. You can add more water if the fruit starts to stick to the bottom of the pan. Add the ginger and/or cinnamon to taste.

2 Meanwhile, make the crumble by gently heating the oil and xylitol in a frying pan. Stir in the oats and toast gently for a few minutes until they start to crispen.

3 Mix in the ground and flaked almonds (or other nuts or seeds) and remove from the heat.

4 Spoon the stewed fruit into bowls and cover with the crumble.

# Juices and smoothies

If your only experience of juices and smoothies is via the concentrated orange juice found in supermarket cartons, or the pasteurised smoothies sold in bottles from chilled counters, you are missing out. Proper juice, fresh from the fruit, has a vitalising quality and a fantastic taste, just as a smoothie straight from the blender has an invigorating freshness that is so much nicer than even the premium brands of smoothies made using pasteurised fruit. It goes without saying that these increasingly fashionable health drinks are also incredibly good sources of vitamins, minerals and phytonutrients – that is, nutrients derived from plants. What is more, they are very easy to digest and absorb, so they are ideal for anyone whose liver is struggling to cope with a toxic overload, or who is ill or recovering from illness or injury. For these reasons we recommend you have a fresh juice or smoothie each day of the nine-day plan (and beyond if you wish), to give your body a regular nutrient burst. Just one word of warning; some fruits are higher in fruit sugars than others: chiefly the tropical fruits like mangoes, lychees, pineapple, bananas, passion fruit and persimmon (Sharon fruit). Juicing extracts the sugars and leaves the fibre, so the sugar is even more rapidly absorbable than by eating the whole fruit. While this is not a problem during the nine-day detox plan, where the focus is on replenishing nutrients and maintaining energy while you omit many other foods, over the long term it is advisable to limit the amount of high-sugar fruits in favour of lower-sugar ones, which release their sugar more slowly to keep blood sugar balanced.

## Equipment

The following items will enable you to make all manner of drinks using every kind of fruit or vegetable imaginable:

- Juice extractor (juicer)

- Citrus press (optional, for citrus fruits like oranges, lemons, grapefruits and limes)

- Hand-held blender or smoothie maker (essential for making smoothies)

Juicers vary in price from the very reasonable to the much more sophisticated models with price tags to match. If you find you are getting in the habit of juicing daily it is worth investing in a good model, as they have stronger motors to withstand regular, heavy use, and extract more juice, and therefore more nutrients, from the fruit.

If you are on a budget, the one item that is essential out of these three is the blender, as you can use this not only to make smoothies but it is also incredibly useful for whizzing soups and the Super Greens Mix that we recommend you add to main meals (see page 122). These can be bought very cheaply indeed.

## Ingredients

The only limit to flavours and combinations of smoothies and juices is your imagination. The possibilities are endless, from the original freshly squeezed OJ to a cooling Caribbean cocktail of coconut milk, banana and mango with crushed ice. The one point that we cannot stress strongly enough, however, is the quality of your ingredients. Where possible, choose organic fruits and vegetables in order to limit your intake of toxic pesticides and waxes that are routinely added to commercial produce. Organic food is also richer in vitamins and minerals than intensively produced fruits and vegetables that have been grown in nutrient-depleted soil and artificially ripened before being stored for long periods. That said, organic apples grown in New Zealand will not contain as much goodness as those that are grown locally, even if they are not strictly speaking organic. The best way to shop is to choose fruits and vegetables that have been grown nearby when they are in season, to cut down on travel time. Supermarkets are increasingly stocking local produce, but other places to look include markets, especially farmers' markets, and local greengrocers, or you may wish to invest in a weekly organic delivery box to keep you well stocked with fresh ingredients.

You should also thoroughly wash all ingredients that do not need peeling. If you are not using organic, try rinsing produce with a 'veggie wash' (available from health-food stores) to remove much of the pesticides and sprays.

## Storage

The whole point of a juice or smoothie is to give your body a short, sharp burst of nutrients. These nutrients are delicate, however, and are depleted by time spent exposed to light, air and heat. Therefore, the sooner you drink your juice or smoothie after processing, the better. If you need to prepare a drink in advance to take to work, then do it that morning rather than the day before, and store it in the fridge or in a chilled container. Add a squeeze of lemon juice to the mixture to prevent it from oxidising and turning brown.

## Fruit

Think beyond the usual choices and add some different colours and flavours to your drinks by using a variety of different ingredients. The more vivid the colour, the higher the nutrient content, and apply the Rainbow Rule to your shopping: choose as many different colours of fruits and vegetables as possible, as each colour indicates a different kind of plant nutrient. Some ideas for your shopping basket include:

Apples

Apricots

Bananas

Berries (including strawberries, raspberries, blueberries, blackberries, blackcurrants, cranberries)

Cherries

Grapefruit, especially pink

Grapes

Guavas

Kiwi fruit

Lemons

Limes

Mangoes

Melons (all types, including watermelon, Galia, honeydew, canteloupe)

Nectarines

Oranges

Papayas

Passion fruit

Peaches

Pears

Pineapples

Plums

Pomegranates

Tangerines, clementines, satsumas

Tomatoes

Limit high-sugar fruits, such as:

Bananas (eat no more frequently than 1 every other day)

Figs

Grapes

Guavas

Kiwis

Lychees

Mangoes

Passion fruit

Persimmon, or Sharon fruit

Pineapples

# Vegetables

Juice from the following vegetables can all be drunk raw, straight from the juicer, even ones like parsnips, which you are more used to seeing served up at Sunday lunch:

Basil

Beetroot

Broccoli (Tenderstem is best)

Cabbage

Carrot

Cauliflower

Celery

Cucumber

Kale

Lettuce

Mint

Parsley

Parsnip

Peppers

Rocket

Root ginger

Baby spinach

Sweet potato

Watercress

## Juices

Here are some classic but delicious juice combinations to get you started and to inspire you to create your own favourites.

# Invigorator

The berries not only sweeten the otherwise too-tart grapefruit but their vibrant colour also provides phyto, or plant-based, nutrients like flavonoids, which help to fight infection. Phytonutrients in grapefruit called limonoids also promote the formation of the detoxifying enzyme glutathione-S-transferase, to help inhibit tumours.

### SERVES 1

1 pink grapefruit
a handful of berries (such as blueberries, raspberries or strawberries)

Push each ingredient through the juicer according to the manufacturer's instructions.

# Skin Nourisher

◼

Simple and sweet, this mixture is extremely good for the complexion thanks to the vitamin C in the apple, from which the body makes collagen, and the beta-carotene in the carrot, which helps disarm free radicals to prevent wrinkles and sun damage. You could also use this as a base to which you could add any other ingredients such as lemon juice and ginger, or celery and cucumber.

**SERVES 1**

1 large apple

1 carrot

Push each ingredient through the juicer according to the manufacturer's instructions.

# C-sharp

◼

This juice is not only an immune-booster that is packed with vitamin C from both the apples and lemon, but the celery is also rich in potassium, which helps to lower blood pressure. If you are not a fan of celery don't worry, its flavour is overpowered by the sweet apple and sharp lemon juice.

**SERVES 1**

1 celery stick

1 large apple

½ lemon (or add the juice separately for a sweeter version)

Push each ingredient through the juicer according to the manufacturer's instructions.

# Stomach Settler

■

All the ingredients in this juice can soothe and heal a troubled digestive tract. Pineapple contains the digestive enzyme bromelain, which helps you breakdown your food and also has strong anti-inflammatory properties. The lemon and ginger add a refreshingly zingy flavour.

**SERVES 1**

1 carrot

1 pear

2 thick slices of fresh pineapple (about a quarter of a medium fruit)

½ lemon (or add the juice separately for a sweeter version)

¼ tsp fresh root ginger

Push each ingredient through the juicer according to the manufacturer's instructions.

# Smoothies

Preparing a smoothie is even easier than a juice, as you simply blend and serve. You can use banana to thicken drinks, but remember that you should not have banana more than every other day, as they are high in starch which will raise blood sugar rapidly. Other ways to add a creamy consistency include coconut milk or non-dairy milks such as unsweetened rice, soya, quinoa, almond and oat milks. Here are a couple of suggestions to get you started.

# Summer Fizz

■

Strawberries and lemons are incredibly rich in vitamin C, and the sweet–sharp flavour combination makes this very refreshing. Make this smoothie in the summer months, however, when strawberries are in season, otherwise you will be paying a premium for flavourless, imported varieties that are of negligible nutritional value. We also recommend naturally sparkling mineral water, as artificially carbonated ones are very abrasive to tooth enamel.

**SERVES 1**

115g (4½oz) (about 5) strawberries

juice of ½ lemon (1 tbsp)

2 tsp xylitol, or to taste

100ml (3½fl oz) sparkling (not carbonated) mineral water

Blend the strawberries and lemon juice until smooth. Stir in the xylitol until it has dissolved then mix in the mineral water.

# Berry Tasty

■

This dairy-free smoothie gets its rich, creamy texture from the tahini (sesame seed paste), which also provides protein to keep your liver detoxing efficiently. Vary the flavour by using strawberries or blueberries instead of raspberries, or a mixture of all three. Xylitol is a safe sugar substitute sourced from plants, which not only does not disrupt blood-sugar levels but is also naturally antibacterial to avoid tooth decay.

**SERVES 1**

75g (3oz) raspberries
1 tbsp tahini
3 tsp xylitol
100ml (3½fl oz) water

Simply blend the ingredients together.

# Watermelon Whizz

■

Its high water content makes watermelon very refreshing and hydrating whereas the deep colour makes it rich in nutrients, including beta-carotene for eye and skin health. The seeds should be kept in as they blend invisibly into the drink yet provide a powerful vitamin E and enzyme punch.

**SERVES 1**

1 medium slice of watermelon, about 200g (7oz) rindless weight

Blend the watermelon flesh, seeds and all, until smooth. Serve with ice or blend the ice with the watermelon for an instant chilled juice.

# Cool Caribbean

■

Bananas are full of the blood-pressure-lowering mineral potassium. They are also full of fibre for aiding the digestion and the fat from the coconut is used as energy rather than being stored as fat. Remember that you should not have more than one banana every other day on the 9-Day Liver Detox, however.

**SERVES 1**

1 banana

a large handful of strawberries

150ml (5fl oz) coconut milk (shake the can before opening, as it separates)

3 ice cubes

Blend all the ingredients together and drink immediately.

# CHAPTER SEVEN

# Your Liver Detox for Life

**W**ell done! You've completed your 9-Day Liver Detox and I hope you are feeling much better. Many people experience such a shift in health, energy, mood and mental clarity that they wonder, 'Should I be eating like this all the time?' Of course, the answer is yes but being this strict all the time is neither easy nor necessary.

The first few days post-detox can be difficult. Don't imagine that you can just go back to your old way of eating and drinking immediately, because your body will rebel. Introduce excluded foods one at a time and slowly, eating only small quantities and chewing well, but don't give up any of the foods you have been eating on the detox diet. Reintroduce the foods in the order I suggest below and if there are any bad reactions, just remove the food you introduced last and move on to the next one. This is the time when you can test whether you are indeed sensitive to any of the excluded foods and to identify which ones they are. Here's how you do it.

## Reintroducing milk

The first food to reintroduce is milk. Have the equivalent of a large glass of it, or cheese or yoghurt, or all of them, on the first day after the nine days' detox. Apart from that, stick to your detox diet. Notice how you feel over the next 48 hours. Particularly notice any digestive symptoms, breathing difficulties or blocked-up nose, headaches, skin itching or joint aches. If you do get such symptoms, there's a good chance you are allergic to milk. Ideally, get yourself tested (see Resources page 172) but certainly keep avoiding milk products.

Few dairy-allergic people react to butter, since it's almost all fat and it's the protein in milk that allergic people react to. Also, most dairy-allergic people also react to goat's and sheep's milk products.

In any event, I don't recommend anyone having dairy products every day. Ideally, keep your milk intake down to 600ml (1 pint) a week and eat plenty of seeds, nuts, beans and lentils as sources of calcium.

## Reintroducing wheat

Wheat is the second food to reintroduce, and with it often comes yeast. On Day 3 after the detox have your first slice of bread – in fact, why not have three? – one or two for breakfast and a nice sandwich for lunch. Notice how you feel over the next 48 hours. Particularly notice any digestive symptoms, bloating, blocked-up nose, headaches, brain fog or mood dips, skin itching or joint aches. If you do get such symptoms, there's a good chance you are allergic to either wheat or yeast. Ideally, get yourself tested (see Resources) but certainly keep avoiding wheat products and yeast for now. By the way, if you seem to be fine on pasta but worse on bread, that's an indication that you are sensitive to yeast.

If you don't react, then my advice is not to have wheat or other gluten grains every day, but choose non-gluten grains instead (see page 35). If you 'rotate' a food, eating it no more than every four days, you are much less likely to become allergic to it.

## Reintroducing alcohol

You might have been inclined to break open the champagne on completing your 9-Day Liver Detox – and why not? You deserve it.

However, the reason I recommend reintroducing wheat and milk first is that alcohol increases your allergic potential by irritating the gut. So I wanted you to have the opportunity to test your sensitivity to wheat and milk before alcohol.

If you want to reintroduce alcohol and measure its effects on you, it is best to choose a yeast-free drink, such as champagne or spirits (a margarita, with fresh lime is probably the best choice). Have a glass or two for three days in a row and notice how it makes you feel. Notice how you feel in the morning, your energy, mental clarity, motivation, mood and digestion. Also, notice your cravings. Personally I would recommend drinking no more than three times a week – ideally no more than one glass or unit – for optimum health. You may find that you feel worse after beer or wine, both of which contain yeast. If so, the chances are you're yeast sensitive.

## Reintroducing meat

It's quite rare to be allergic to meat but it can happen, so watch your symptoms over the next three days after your detox, noting particularly any digestive symptoms. Meat is tough on the digestive system, particularly after a two-week break, so eat only a small amount at the first meal. Start with chicken and build up to red meats slowly. Meat will alter the acid–alkaline balance in your body for the worse, so don't decrease the fruits and vegetables, as they will counter the effect of the meat.

## Reintroducing caffeine

Many people experience so much more energy that they simply don't need the short-term energy boost that caffeine gives, and hence don't crave it. If so, the best course of action is to stay caffeine-free. If, on the other hand, you want to test its effects, have a strong cup of coffee and notice how it makes you feel. Notice your mood, aggression, mental clarity and cravings the next day. Caffeine is very addictive and once you start having it every day you'll crave it every day. However, having the odd cup of tea or infrequent coffee is not a big deal, as long as it doesn't become habit-forming. Certainly don't exceed one coffee a day, two cups of tea or three green teas on a regular basis. It's good to give caffeine a total break every now and then just to make sure you're not getting dependent on it.

# Reintroducing bad fats and fried food

... but it's better if you don't. Generally it's best to stay away from fried foods and processed fat as they damage your cell membranes, preventing nutrients from getting in and waste products from being removed. However, they are neither addictive nor cause allergic reactions. So, my advice is generally to avoid deep-fried foods and junk food high in processed or hydrogenated fats. However, the odd indulgence is not going to kill you.

# How to use your liver detox for life

If you've achieved what you set out to achieve and your detox score (see page 77) has dropped substantially then the question is how to make the habits you have learned into your habits for life.

My advice is to follow the 80/20 rule. That is, stick to the detox-diet principles for 80 per cent of the time and be less strict on yourself 20 per cent of the time.

In practical terms what this means is:

- Drink at least 1 litre (1¾ pints), or six glasses, of water every day

- Have a superfood twice a day

- Have three servings of antioxidant-rich foods a day, including cruciferous vegetables

- Eat wheat and milk products no more than once every four days

- Have alcohol or caffeinated drinks every five days (that means six times a month)

- Have seeds six days out of seven

- Take supplements every day

# Supplements for super-health

Once you've completed your 9-Day Liver Detox, which you may wish to extend to 30 days, there is no need to keep taking the additional supplements, but every reason to continue with the basics, which are:

- A high potency multivitamin and mineral

- One to two grams of vitamin C, plus bioflavonoids found in berry extracts

- Essential omega-3 (EPA and DHA) and omega-6 (GLA) fats

Good multivitamins state on the pack, 'take twice a day' not only because you can't get enough in a single tablet unless you make it a horse pill but also because taking supplements twice a day is more effective. This is because the water-soluble vitamins B and C are only available in the body for up to six hours. So, your basic daily supplement programme should look like the following. Remember to take supplements every day at breakfast and lunchtime:

|  | Dosage | |
| --- | --- | --- |
|  | **Breakfast** | **Lunch** |
| High-potency multivitamin | 1 | 1 |
| Vitamin C | 1 | 1 |
| Essential fats (DHA, GLA and EPA) | 1 | |

We hope that your experiences during the 9-Day Liver Detox have both helped you regain health and also helped you to learn what kind of diet and lifestyle suit you best, and that it has given you the tools and the inspiration to stick to it. If you ever do feel like you are going downhill, make a resolution to do another 9-Day Liver Detox and get your health back on track!

# Notes

## Chapter 1

1 Kaya, H., Koc, A., Sogut, S., Duru, M., Yilmaz, H.R., Uz, E., Durgut, R., 'The protective effect of N-acetylcysteine against cyclosporine A-induced hepatotoxicity in rats', *Journal of Applied Toxicology*, (27 April 2007), epub ahead of print. Ruffmann, R *et al.*, 'GSH rescue by N-acetylcysteine', *Klin. Wochenschr* Vol. 69 (1991), pp. 857–62; Woo, O, *et al.*, 'Shorter duration of oral N-acetylcysteine therapy for acute acetaminophen overdose', *Annals of Emergency Medicine*, Vol. 35 (4) (April 2000), pp. 363–8; Flora, S, 'Arsenic-induced oxidative stress and its reversibility following combined administration of N-acetyl cysteine and Meso 2, 3-dimercaptosuccinic acid in rats', *Clinical and Experimental Pharmacology and Physiology*, Vol 26 (11) (November 1999), pp. 865–9; Makin, A, *et al.*, '7-year experience of severe acetaminophen-induced hepatotoxicity (1987–1993)', *Gastroenterology*, Vol. 109 (6) (December 1995), pp. 1907–16; Villa, P, and Ghezzi, P, 'Effect of N-acetylcysteine on sepsis in mice', *European Journal of Pharmacology*, Vol. 292 (3-4) (March 1995), pp. 341–4.

2 Weber, C., Jakobsen, T.S., Mortensen, S.A., Paulsen, G., Holmer, G., 'Effect of dietary coenzyme Q10 as an antioxidant in human plasma', *Molecular Aspects of Medicine*; 15 (1994), Suppl: S97–102.

3 *Modern Nutrition in Health & Disease*, 8th edn; pp. 432–48 and Schwedhelm, E., Maas, R., Troost, R., Boger, R.H., 'Clinical pharmacokinetics of anti-oxidants and their impact on systemic oxidative stress', *Clinical Pharmacokinetics*, Vol. 42(5) (2003), pp. 437–59.

4 *Modern Nutrition in Health & Disease*, 8th edn; pp. 326–41 and Schwedhelm, E., Maas, R., Troost, R., Boger, R.H., 'Clinical pharmacokinetics of anti-oxidants and their impact on systemic oxidative stress', *Clinical Pharmacokinetics*, Vol. 42(5) (2003), pp. 437–59 and Van Haaften, R.I., Haenen, G.R., Evelo, C.T., Bast, A., 'Effect of vitamin E on glutathione-

dependent enzymes', *Drug Metabolism Reviews*, Vol. 35(2–3) (May–August 2003), pp. 215–53.

5 Schwedhelm, E., Maas, R., Troost, R., Boger, R.H., 'Clinical pharmacokinetics of antioxidants and their impact on systemic oxidative stress', *Clinical Pharmacokinetics*, Vol. 42(5): (2003) pp. 437–59.

6 Schwedhelm, E., Maas, R., Troost, R., Boger, R.H., 'Clinical pharmacokinetics of antioxidants and their impact on systemic oxidative stress', *Clinical Pharmacokinetics*, Vol. 42(5) (2003), pp. 437–59.

7 Touvier, M., Kesse, E., Clavel-Chapelon, F., Boutron-Ruault, M.C., 'Dual association of beta-carotene with risk of tobacco-related cancers in a cohort of French women', *Journal of the National Cancer Institute*, Vol. 97(18) (21 September 2005), pp. 1338–44 and Virtamo, J., Pietinen, P., Huttunen, J.K., Korhonen, P., Malila, N., Virtanen, M.J., Albanes, D., Taylor, P.R., Albert, P., ATBC Study Group, 'Incidence of cancer and mortality following alpha-tocopherol and beta-carotene supplementation: a postintervention follow-up', *Journal of the American Medical Association*, Vol. 290(4) (23 July 2003), pp. 476–85.

8 Gaziano, J.M., 'Vitamin E and cardiovascular disease: observational studies', *Annals of the New York Academy of Science*, 1031 (Dec 2004), pp. 280–91 and McQueen, M.J., Lonn, E., Gerstein, H.C., Bosch, J., Yusuf, S., 'The HOPE (Heart Outcomes Prevention Evaluation) Study and its consequences', *Scandinavian Journal of Clinical and Laboratory Investigation*, 240 (2005), pp. 143–56.

9 Yoshida, M., Katashima, S., Ando, J., Tanaka, T., Uematsu, F., Nakae, D., Maekawa, A., 'Dietary indole-3-carbinol promotes endometrial adeno-carcinoma development in rats initiated with N-ethyl-N'-nitro-N-nitroso-guanidine, with induction of cytochrome P450s in the liver and consequent modulation of estrogen metabolism', *Carcinogenesis*, Vol. 25(11) (November 2004), pp. 2257–64, epub (7 July 2004).

10 Moon, Y.J., Wang, X., Morris, M.E., 'Dietary flavonoids: effects on xenobiotic and carcinogen metabolism', *Toxicology In Vitro*, Vol. 20(2) (March 2006), pp. 187–210, epub 11 November 2005, Review, and Hodek, P., Trefil, P., Stiborova, M., 'Flavonoids-potent and versatile biologically active compounds interacting with cytochromes P450', *Chemical and Biological Interactions*, Vol. 139(1) (22 January 2002), pp. 1–21.

11 Kay, C.D., Holub, B.J., 'The effect of wild blueberry (*Vaccinium angustifolium*) consumption on postprandial serum antioxidant status in human subjects', *Journal of Agricultural and Food Chemistry*, Vol. 50(26) (18 December 2002), pp. 7731–7.

12 Morand, C., Crespy, V., Manach, C., Besson, C., Demigne, C., Remesy, C., 'Plasma metabolites of quercetin and their antioxidant properties',

*American Journal of Physiology* (1998); 275 (1 Pt 2): R212–9 and de Groot, H., Rauen, U., 'Tissue injury by reactive oxygen species and the protective effects of flavonoids', *Fundamentals of Clinical Pharmacology*, Vol. 12(3), (1998) pp. 249–55.

13  Cody, V., Middleton, E., and Harborne, J.B., *Plant Flavonoids in Biology and Medicine II*, Alan R. Lis Inc. (1988), pp. 135–8.

14  Hruby, K., Csomos, G., Fuhrmann, M., Thaler, H., 'Chemotherapy of Amanita phalloides poisoning with intravenous silibinin', *Human Toxicology* 2 (1983), pp. 183–95, and Salmi, H.A., Sarna, S., 'Effect of silymarin on chemical, functional, and morphological alterations of the liver. A double-blind controlled study', *Scandinavian Journal of Gastroenterology*, Vol. 17(4) (1982), pp. 517–21 and *Virchows Archive B – Cell Pathology Including Molecular Pathology*, 64 (1993), pp. 259–63 and *Gastroenterology* 109 (1995), pp. 1941–49 and Kropacova, K., Misurova, E., Hakova, H., 'Protective and therapeutic effect of silymarin on the development of latent liver damage', *Radiatsionnaia biologiia, radioecologiia*, 38 (1998), pp. 411–15; Campos R, *et al.*, 'Silybin dihemisuccinate protects against glutathione depletion and lipid peroxidation induced by acetaminophen on rat liver', *Planta Med*, Vol. 55 (1989), pp. 417–9.

15  Dwivedi, C., Heck, W.J., Downie, A.A., Larroya, S., Webb, T.E., 'Effect of calcium glucarate on beta-glucuronidase activity and glucarate content of certain vegetables and fruits', *Biochemical Medicine and Metabolic Biology*, Vol. 43(2) (1990) pp. 83–92 and Nijhoff, W.A., Mulder, T.P., Verhagen, H., van Poppel, G., Peters, W.H., 'Effects of consumption of Brussels sprouts on plasma and urinary glutathione S-transferase class-alpha and -pi in humans', *Carcinogenesis*, Vol. 16(4) (April 1995), pp. 955–7.

16  Khashab, M., Tector, A.J., Kwo, P.Y., 'Epidemiology of acute liver failure', *Current Gastroenterology Reports*, Vol. 9(1) (March 2007), pp. 66–73.

17  Biewenga, G, et al., 'The pharmacology of the antioxidant lipoic acid', *General Pharmacology*, Vol. 29 (September 1997), pp. 315–31; Kanna, S, *et al.*, 'Alpha lipoic acid supplementation: tissue glutathione homeostasis at rest and after exercise', *Journal of Applied Physiology*, Vol. 86 (4) (April 1999), pp. 1191–6; Han, D, et al., 'Lipoic acid increases de novo synthesis of cellular glutathione by improving cysteine utilization', *Biofactors*, Vol. 6 (3) (1997), pp. 321–8; Bustamente, J, et al., 'Alpha lipoic acid in liver metabolism and disease', *Free Radical Biology and Medicine*, Vol. 24 (6) (April 1998), pp. 1023–39.

## Chapter 2

1  Hourigan, C.S., 'The molecular basis of celiac disease', *Clinical and Experimental Medicine*, Vol. 6(2) 2006, pp. 53–9.

2  Sandiford, C.P., *et al.*, 'Identification of the major water/salt insoluble wheat proteins involved in cereal hypersensitivity', *Clinical and Experimental Allergy*, Vol. 27 (1997), pp. 1120–9

3  Stoersrud, S., *et al.*, 'Adult coeliac disease patients do tolerate large amounts of oats', *European Journal of Clinical Nutrition*, Vol. 57 (2003), pp. 163–9 and Hoegberg, L., *et al.*, 'Oats to children with newly diagnosed coeliac disease: a randomised double blind study', *Gut*, Vol. 54 (2004), pp. 645–54.

4  Torres, M.I., Lopez Casado, M.A., Rios, A., 'New aspects in celiac disease', *World Journal of Gastroenterology* Vol. 13(8) (28 February 2007), pp. 1156–61.

5  http://osiris.sunderland.ac.uk/autism/

6  http://www.greatplainslaboratory.com/russian/glutencasein.html and www.osiris.sunderland.ac.uk/autism/aru.htm

7  US National Institutes of Health (http://digestive.niddk.nih.gov/diseases/pubs/lactoseintolerance/)

8  LeRoith, D., Roberts Jr, C.T., 'The insulin-like growth factor system and cancer', *Cancer Letters*, Vol. 195(2) (10 June 2003), pp. 127–37. Review.

9  Juliano, L.M., Griffiths, R.R., 'A critical review of caffeine withdrawal: empirical validation of symptoms and signs, incidence, severity, and associated features', *Psychopharmacology* (Berl), Vol. 176(1) (October 2004), pp. 1–29.

10  Rogers, P.J., Heatherley, S.V., Hayward, R.C., Seers, H.E., Hill, J., Kane, M., *Psychopharmacology* (Berl), 'Effects of caffeine and caffeine withdrawal on mood and cognitive performance degraded by sleep restriction', Vol. 179(4) (June 2005), pp. 742–52.

11  Gilliland, K. and Adress, D., 'Ad lib caffeine consumption, symptoms of caffeinism, and academic performance', *American Journal of Psychiatry*, Vol. 138(4), (1981) pp. 512–14.

12  Institute for Optimum Nutrition, ONUK Survey, 2004. See www.ion.ac.uk

13  Vlachopoulos, C., Panagiotakos, D., Ioakeimidis, N., Dima, I., Stefanadis, C., 'Chronic coffee consumption has a detrimental effect on aortic stiffness and wave reflections', *American Journal of Clinical Nutrition*, Vol. 81(6) (June 2005), pp. 1307–12.

14  Refsum, H., *et al.*, 'The Hordaland Homocysteine Study – A Community-Based Study of Homocysteine, its Determinants, and Associations with Disease 1', *Journal of Nutrition*, 136 (2006), pp. 1731S–1740S.

15  A 50 per cent higher level of one of the markers (known as Interleukin 6), a 30 per cent higher level of another (known as C-reactive protein) and a 28 per cent higher level of a third (known as TNF) compared to non-coffee

consumers. Zampelas, A., Panagiotakos, D.B., Pitsavos, C., Chrysohoou, C., Stefanadis, C., 'Associations between coffee consumption and inflammatory markers in healthy persons: the ATTICA study', *American Journal of Clinical Nutrition*, Vol. 80(4) (October 2004), pp. 862-7.

16 Shilo, L., Sabbah, H., Hadari, R., Kovatz, S., Weinberg, U., Dolev, S., Dagan, Y., Shenkman, L., 'The effects of coffee consumption on sleep and melatonin secretion', *Sleep Medicine*, (May 2002), Vol. 3(3), pp. 271-3.

17 Waluga, M., Hartleb, M.,'Alcoholic liver disease', *Wiadomosci Lekarskie*. Vol. 56(1-2) (2003), pp. 61-70, Review, and Bae, K.S., Yoo, K., Cho, Y.K., Shim, K.N., Jung, S.A., Moon, I.H., 'The short term prognosis in alcoholic liver disease with metabolic acidosis', *Korean Journal of Hepatology*, Vol. 10(2), (June 2004), pp. 117-24.

18 'Food, Nutrition and the Prevention of Cancer: a Global Perspective', World Cancer Research Fund/American Institute for Cancer Research, 1997, chapter 5.5.

## Chapter 3

1 Thomas, B. (ed.), *Manual of Dietetic Practice*, 3rd edn, Blackwell Publishing, 2001.

2 Kleiner, S.M., 'Water: an essential but overlooked nutrient', *Journal of the American Dietetic Association*, Vol. 99(2) (1999), pp. 200-6.

3 Thomas, B. (ed.), *Manual of Dietetic Practice*, 3rd edn, Blackwell Publishing, 2001.

4 Batmanghelidj, F., *Your Body's Many Cries For Water*, Tagman Press, 1992.

5 Durga, J., *et al.*, 'Effect of a 3-year folic acid supplementation on cognitive function in older adults in the FACIT trial: a randomised, double blind, controlled trial', *The Lancet*, Vol. 369 (9557), (2007), pp. 208-16.

6 Block, G., 'Epidemiologic evidence regarding vitamin C and cancer', *American Journal of Clinical Nutrition*, Vol. 54(6 Suppl) (December 1991), pp. 1310S-1314S.

7 Nijhoff, W., *et al.*, 'Effects of consumption of Brussels sprouts on intestinal and lymphocytic glutathione S-transferases in humans', *Carcinogenisis*, Vol. 16(9) (1995), pp. 2125-8.

# Resources

## Patrick Holford organisations

**The Holford Diet Club**, called Zest4Life, provides advice and support for weight loss through a series of weekly meetings, including many of the detox principles. For more information, visit www.holforddiet.com

**The Institute for Optimum Nutrition** (ION) offers a three-year foundation degree course in nutritional therapy that includes training in the optimum nutrition approach to mental health. There is a clinic, a list of nutrition practitioners across the UK and overseas, an information service and a quarterly journal, *Optimum Nutrition*.

Contact ION at Avalon House, 72 Lower Mortlake Road, Richmond TW9 2JY, UK, or call +44 (0) 870 979 1122 or visit www.ion.ac.uk.

**To find a nutritional therapist near you** visit www.patrickholford. com and click on 'consultations'.

## Water filters

There are many water filters on the market. One of the best is offered by The Fresh Water Filter Company, who produce mains-attached water-filtering units using gravity rather than reverse osmosis (which can filter out some useful minerals as well). You can buy a whole-house filter or an under-sink version.

For details contact Health Products for Life on +44 (0)2-8874 8038 or go to www.healthproductsforlife.com

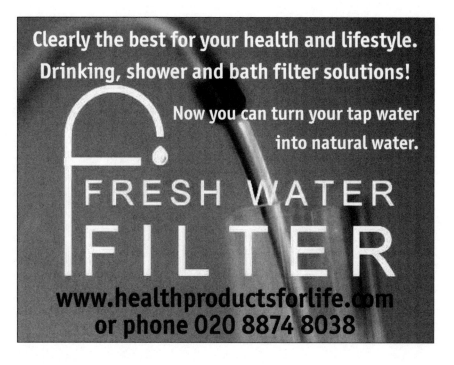
## Psychocalisthenics

**Psychocalisthenics** is an exercise system that takes less than 20 minutes a day, and develops strength, suppleness and stamina and generates vital energy. The best way to learn it is to do the Psychocalisthenics training. See www.patrickholford.com (seminars) for details on this or call +44 (0) 20 8871 2949. Also available in the book *Master Level Exercise: Psychocalisthenics* and on the Psychocalisthenics CD and DVD. For further information, see www.pcals.com

## Supplements

**Health Products for Life** is an online shop for a range of health-promoting products including the AGE antioxidant formula, digestive enzymes, glutamine powder and the Optimum Nutrition Pack, a daily sachet containing an optimum nutrition multivitamin, vitamin C and essential fats. They also have a 9-Day Pack to support your Detox diet (see www.healthproductforlife.com/ninedaypack).

Visit www.healthproductsforlife.com or call +44 (0)20 8874 8038.

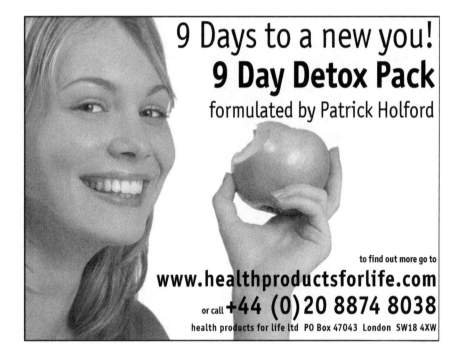
## Tests

**Liver Detoxification Profile** Contact Individual Wellbeing Laboratories on +44 (0)20 8336 7750 or go to www.iwdl.net. This urine test identifies how effective your body's Phase-1 and Phase-2 detoxification is. This helps identify which nutrients are important to include in your Detox diet, and which substances are especially important for you to avoid. This test is also available from www.healthproductsforlife.com or call +44 (0) 20 8874 8038.

**Food allergies or sensitivities** Contact YorkTest Laboratories on FREE-POST NEA5, 243 York, YO19 5ZZ, or telephone 0800 074 6185, or go to www.yorktest.com. YorkTest Laboratories offer a home-test kit for food allergy (IgG ELISA) and homocysteine testing. With this you can take your own pinprick blood sample and return it to the lab for analysis. This test identifies if you have any food allergies to any of 113 foods, including gluten and gliadin. Food allergy testing is best done under the guidance of a nutritional therapist. This test is also available from www.healthproductsforlife.com or call +44 (0) 20 8874 8038.

To help interpret the results of any of these tests, you may wish to contact one of my highly trained **nutritional therapists**. Go to my web-site www.patrickholford.com to find a nutritional therapist near you.

**Yoga** If you would like to try yoga as a form of stretching exercise and relaxation look at the website for The British Wheel of Yoga www. bwy.org.uk to find a class with a trained teacher near you.

# Recommended Reading List

Holford, Patrick, *The New Optimum Bible*, Piatkus, 2005

Holford, Patrick, *The Holford Low-GL Diet*, Piatkus, 2004

Holford, Patrick and McDonald Joyce, Fiona, *The Holford Low-GL Diet Cookbook*, Piatkus, 2005

Holford, Patrick, *Improve Your Digestion*, Piatkus Books, 1999

MacDonald Baker, Sidney, *Detoxification and Healing*, McGraw-Hill, 2003

Lipski, Elizabeth, *Digestive Wellness*, Keats Publishing, 1996

Bland, Jeffrey, *The 20-Day Rejuvenation Diet Program*, Keats Publishing, 1997

# Index

Page numbers in **bold** refer to diagrams, page numbers in *italics* refer to information in tables.

# Index of Recipes

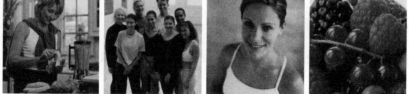
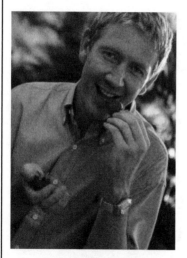